INTANGIBLE CULTURAL HERITAGE OF INDIA

INTANGIBLE CULTURAL HERITAGE OF INDIA (VOL. II)

ETHNO-MEDICINE IN INDIA

A Selective Bibliography

Kamal Kant Misra
Mohammad Rehan
Ravindra K. Gupta

Indira Gandhi Rashtriya Manav Sangrahalaya
(National Museum of Mankind)
Bhopal

GYAN

GYAN PUBLISHING HOUSE

First Published - 2013

Cataloguing in Publication (CIP) data:

Misra, K.K. [et al.]
Intangible Cultural Heritage of India: A Selective Bibliography/by K.K. Misra, Ravindra K. Gupta and Mohammad Rehan - New Delhi : Gyan Publishing House, 2013.

2v.

Content: v.1. Indian Religious Practices (Fairs, Festivals, Customs, Beliefs, Ceremonies, Rites, Rituals, Manners, Traditions)- v. 2. Ethno-medicine in India.

I. Title II. Gupta, Ravindra K. III. Mohammad Rehan
615.88
ISBN : 978-81-212-1189-5
Published by :
Gyan Publishing House
23, Main Ansari Road, Daryaganj
New Delhi-110002
Phones : 23282060, 23261060
Fax : 011-23285914
E-mail: books@gyanbooks.com
Website: www.gyanbooks.com

and

Indira Gandhi Rashtriya Manav Sangrahalaya
Shamla Hills, Bhopal
Phones : 0755-2661290, 2661319
Fax : 91-755-2661458
E-mail : directorigrms@gmail.com

Laser Typesetting : Rudra Computer Graphics, Delhi
Printed at : Salasar Imaging System, Delhi

Contents

Preface

A well-organized information system is a prerequisite for the growth and development of any discipline. It can efficiently and effectively serve the needs of the seeker of nascent information. Bibliography is one such useful information system, as it acquaints the scholars and research workers with the work already done in the past on a particular subject, region or place, author, etc. Quick and easy access to information is vital to the development of various fields of knowledge. Therefore, it is essential that relevant information be brought to the attention of the professionals, administrators, and researchers who have urgent need of it. In this respect, bibliography plays an important role. There was a time in the past, when it was possible for a scholar to keep herself/himself uptodate and well informed on current literature in the field of interest. But due to the increase in the amount of literature available, it has become more and more difficult for him/her to do so. But for bibliography even a scholar faced with such a vast amount of literature would lose his/her way, wasting much time before he/she is able to read even a part of what he/she is required to study.

Much has been written on Indian ethno-medicine and the references are many and distributed over numerous journals, monographs, memoirs, internet database and other publications that are not easily accessible to research workers and the seekers of information. Keeping in view these facts, it was considered useful to compile a bibliography on the subject.

This bibliography on 'Ethno-medicine of India' indexes 2034 monographs (books), Journal articles, research papers, thesis, notes, etc. The bibliography is aimed at covering scholarly literature on Ethno-medicine and related fields.

In the compilation of this comprehensive bibliography, varieties of sources have been used. They can be broadly classified as:

(a) Individual Journals (b) Monographs (books)

(c) Bibliographies (e) INTERNET database

(d) Indexing/ Abstracting services (Local and International)

Structure of the Bibliography

Each entry in the bibliography contains information:

Books : Name of Author/editor (Surname, forename), Title of book (in double inverted comma), Place of publication, Name of publisher, Year of publication, and total pages of book.

Example: Pandey, R. P. "Pre-historic archaeology of Madhya Pradesh". New Delhi, Sandeep Prakashan, 1987, p. 296.

Journal Article: Name of Author (Surname, forename), Title (in double inverted comma), Name of Journals (in *Italic*), Volume No., Issue No., Year, and the pages.

Example: Mathpal, Y. "Rock art sites in India and problems of their preservation and management". *Purakala*, Vol. 2, No. 1, 1991, pp. 22-23.

The bibliography consists of full entries arranged alphabetically under authors. Each entry has been serially numbered. To facilitate quick references from any desired viewpoint three alphabetical indices, *vis.*, Subject/Keyword Index, and Title Index, referring to the text by the serial number, have been appended.

We sincerely hope that this bibliography would be useful for scientists, research scholars, and other personnel related to the field of ethno-medicine.

Kamal Kant Misra

Ravindra Kumar Gupta

Mohammad Rehan

Abbreviation used

A.P.	:	Andhra Pradesh
AIOC	:	All India Oriental Congress
Annon.	:	Anonymous
CRM	:	Cultural Resource Management
D.C.R.I	:	Deccan College and Research Centre
GPS	:	Global Positioning System.
IAHC	:	Indian Art History Congress
IAR	:	Indian Anthropological Review
IGNCA	:	Indira Gandhi National Centre for Arts
IGRMS	:	Indira Gandhi Rasstriya Manav Sangrahalaya
JAOS	:	Journal of the American Oriental Society
JRASB	:	Journal of Asiatic Society of Bengal
M. P.	:	Madhya Pradesh
Ph.D.	:	Doctor in Philosophy
PILC	:	Journal of Dravidic Studies
T. N.	:	Tamil Nadu
U.P.	:	Uttar Pradesh
UGC	:	University Grant Commission
UNESCO	:	United Nations Educational, Scientific and Cultural Organization

List of Journals

1. **Acta Botanica Indica**: Published by the Society for Advancement of Botany, Meerut (India).
2. **Adibasi:** Quarterly Journal of Tribal and Harijan Research-cum-Training Inst, Bhubaneswar
3. **Advances in Plant Sciences**: A biannual journal of the Academy of Plant Sciences, India (APSI) was established in 1987 to promote awareness, advancement and to disseminate knowledge on commercial and scientific aspects of plants to project and importance of conservation and propagation of Indian plants and to further strengthen the plant sciences fraternity.
4. **African journal of Traditional, Complementary and Alternative Medicines**: The African Journal of Traditional, Complementary and Alternative medicines (AJTCAM), a new broad-based journal, is founded on two key tenets: To publish exciting research in all areas of applied medicinal plants, Traditional medicines, Complementary Alternative Medicines, food and agricultural technologies, and promotion of healthy use of medicinal products. Secondly, to provide the most rapid turn-around time possible for reviewing and publishing, and to disseminate the articles freely for teaching and reference purposes. All articles published in AJTCAM are peer-reviewed.
5. **American Anthropologist**: American Anthropologist is the flagship journal of the American Anthropological Association and is published on a quarterly basis. American Anthropologist follows the mission statement and goals of the

American Anthropological Association by advancing anthropology as a discipline that studies humankind in all its aspects, involving archaeological, biological, ethnological, and linguistic research. It also attempts to further the professional interests of anthropologists by disseminating anthropological knowledge and illuminating its relevance to human problems.

6. **American Ethnologist**: Published by Journal of the American Ethnological Society, concerned with ethnology in the term's broadest sense. Articles published in the journal explore connections between ethnographic specificity and theoretical originality, and convey the relevance of the ethnographic imagination to the contemporary world. As a flagship journal for social and cultural anthropology, American Ethnologist is well positioned to disseminate work that roams across an extraordinary variety of theoretical approaches, methods, and points of view.
7. **American Sociological Review**: The American Sociological Review is the flagship journal of the American Sociological Association (ASA). The ASA founded this journal in 1936 (Vol. 1) with the mission to publish original works of interest to the sociology discipline in general, new theoretical development, result of research that advance our understanding of fundamental social process, and important methodological innovations.
8. **Ancient Science of Life**: Ancient Science of Life, is the oldest peer reviewed scientific journal in Ayurveda which publishes full-length original papers and reviews on Ayurveda, allied disciplines and all forms of traditional medicines.
9. **Angarag:** All the Visual matters: A biyearly publication by Gurudebaprasad Dance Institute, Bhubaneswar, India,
10. **Annals of Internal medicine**: Established in 1927 by the American College of Physicians (ACP), Annals of Internal Medicine is the premier internal medicine journal. Annals of Internal Medicine's mission is to promote excellence in medicine, enable physicians and other health care professionals to be well informed members of the medical community and society, advance standards in the conduct and reporting of medical research, and contribute to improving the health of people worldwide.

11. **Anthropology Today**: Anthropology Today is a bimonthly publication which aims to provide a forum for the application of anthropological analysis to public and topical issues, while reflecting the breadth of interests within the discipline of anthropology.

12. **Antiquity:** Antiquity, a quarterly, peer-reviewed journal of archaeology, founded by O.G.S. Crawford in 1927, is owned by the Antiquity Trust, a registered charity. The Trustees of the Antiquity Trust are Graeme Barker, Warwick Bray, Robin Coningham, Barry Cunliffe, Chris Gosden, Anthony Harding, Paul Mellars, Colin Renfew and Stephen Shennan. The Directors of Antiquity Publications Ltd., owned by the Antiquity Trust and responsible for producing Antiquity are Martin Carver, Chris Evans, Roger Guthrie, Martin Millett, Nicky Milner, Cameron Petrie, Mike Pitts and Andrew Rogerson.

13. **Archives of Applied Science Research:** (Available online at www.scholarsresearchlibrary.com)

14. **Arogya: Journal of Health Science: Edited** by T N Pattabiraman, Kasturba Gandhi Medical College Trust, Andhra Pradesh.

15. **Aryavaidyan**: Aryavaidyan the quarterly journal of Arya Vaidya Sala, Kottakkal is a publication entirely devoted to the cause of Ayurveda and allied subjects for which Vaidyaratnam P. S. Varier, who founded this institution had dedicated everything.

16. **Asian Agri-History**: Published by the Asian Agri-History Foundation (AAHF), a non-profit trust, was established and registered in 1994 to facilitate dissemination of information on agricultural history published every quarter.

17. **Asian Journal of Traditional Medicines**: AJTM has been founded jointly by Shenyang Pharmaceutical University and Herbal Font Pharmaceutical Limited. The journal is published by Hong Kong Asiamed Publishing House, bimonthly in English, and is available outside China.

18. **Biodiversity and Conservation**: Biodiversity and Conservation is an international journal that publishes articles on all aspects of biological diversity-its description, analysis and conservation, and its controlled rational use by

humankind. The scope of Biodiversity and Conservation is wide and multidisciplinary, and embraces all life-forms. Biodiversity and Conservation is published monthly by Springer.

19. **Botanical Museum leaflets, Harvard University:** Published by Botanical Museum. Cambridge, Massachusetts

20. **Bryologist:** The American Bryological and Lichenological Society Inc., Society publishes a quarterly journal distributed world-wide. The first issue of The Bryologist was published in 1898, with the formation of the Society.

21. **Bulletin of Indian Institute of History of Medicine (BIIHM)**: A Biannual Journals published for the Central Council for Research in Ayurveda & Siddha, New Delhi.

22. **Bulletin of Medico-Ethno-botanical Research**: Quarterly published by Central Council for Research in Ayurveda & Siddha, New Delhi

23. **Bulletin of Meghalaya Science Society: Published by** Meghalaya Science Society, North-Eastern Hill University, Shillong, Meghalaya, India

24. **Bulletin of National Institute of Science of India**: The National Institute of Sciences of India, now the Indian National Science Academy, New Delhi (INSA) is a premier science Academy in the country, plays crucial role in promoting, recognizing and rewarding excellence. Another important task is to publish journals, organize scientific discussions and bring out proceedings and monographs.

25. **Bulletin of Regional Research Laboratory, Jammu:** A publication of Regional Research Laboratory, Jammu.

26. **Bulletin of the Bihar Tribal Research Institute**: Published by Bihar Tribal Research Institute, Bihar Tribal Research Institute, Ranchi, India

27. **Bulletin of the Botanical Survey of India**: Published by Botanical Survey of India, Kolkata

28. **Bulletin of the Deccan College Research Institute**: The Deccan College in Pune is the third oldest educational institution in the country. In recognition of the excellence achieved by the Institute both in teaching and research, the H.R.D. Ministry, Government of India, awarded it the status of a Deemed University on 5th March 1990.

29. **Bulletin of the Department of Anthropology, Guwahati University:** Published by the Guwahati University, Department of the Anthropology, Guwahati.
30. **Bulletin of the Department of Anthropology**: Published by the Department of Anthropology, Indian Museum Calcutta.
31. **Bulletin of the Tribal Research and Development Institute:** (TRI), Bhopal, Madhya Pradesh
32. **Canadian Family Physician**: Canadian Family Physician (CFP), a peer-reviewed medical journal, is the official publication of the College of Family Physicians of Canada.
33. **CCRAS Newsletter**: The Central Council for Research in Ayurvedic Sciences (CCRAS) is an autonomous body of the department of AYUSH (Ayurveda, Yoga and Naturopathy, Unani, Siddha and Homeopathy), Ministry of Health and Family Welfare, Government of India.
34. **Chaumasa**: Adivasi Lok Kala has been publishing Choumasa (in Hindi), a quarterly magazine centered on folk arts, music, literature and culture since 1983. The magazine serves as a significant source of rare materials on the various aspects of tribal culture and their art forms.
35. **Current Science**: The Current Science is a science journal cum Magazine started in 1932. It is published by Current Science Association in collaboration with the Indian Academy of Sciences, Bangalore. The bi- monthly issue of current science has articles related to all science disciplines and general views about science and scientific community/ development.
36. **Discover India**: Discover India, India's premium travel and culture magazine was launched in 1988 by Media Transasia India Limited in active cooperation with the Ministry of Tourism, Government of India, with a view to cater primarily to the inbound tourist. Discover India Magazine is a travel magazine full of insights about India.
37. **Down to Earth:** Society for Environmental Communications started India's only science and environment fortnightly, Down To Earth (DTE). Over the years the magazine has informed and inspired people about environmental threats facing India and the world.

38. **Drugs Himalayan Research and Development:**

39. **Eastern Anthropologist**: The Eastern Anthropologist is a refereed, quarterly journal of the Ethnographic and Folk Culture Society. Journal Founded in 1947 by Dr. D.N. Majumdar, Published by Serial Publications on behalf of Ethnographic and Folk culture Society, Lucknow, India.

40. **Economic and Political Weekly**: The Economic and Political Weekly, published by Sameeksha Trust, Mumbai, registered charitable trust, is the only social science journal of its kind in the world. Where other reputed journals publish either only comments on contemporary affairs or research papers, EPW is unique in that week it publishes analysis of contemporary affairs side by side with academic papers in the social sciences.

41. **Economic Botany**: Economic Botany is a quarterly journal published by The New York Botanical Garden for the Society for Economic Botany. Interdisciplinary in scope, Economic Botany bridges the gap between pure and applied botany by focusing on the uses of plants by people.

42. **Environmental Ethics:** An Interdisciplinary Journal Dedicated to the Philosophical Aspects of Environmental Problems. The Center for Environmental Philosophy was created by the board of directors of Environmental Philosophy, Inc., a nonprofit corporation of the State of New Mexico. It is the product of a number of activities begun with the creation of the journal Environmental Ethics.

43. **Ethnobotanical Leafletts**: Ethnobotanical Leaflets is an international online journal that aims to promote the exchange of original knowledge and research in any area of ethnobotany and to disseminate information and ideas that may help to sustainable management of resources.

44. **Ethnology:** Ethnology is published quarterly with an additional issues published in October by the University of Pittsburg, Pittsburg and supported jointly by the Anthropology and University Library System.

45. **Ethnomedizin** (Ethnomedicine): Journal/ Newspaper in German, English.

46. **Folklore**: The Folklore devoted to the cause of the Indian Folklore Society, Calcutta. It provides clear authoritative

coverage of the issues that matter in the folklore and folk life research.

47. **Health and Population Perspectives and Issues**: Published by National Institute of Health and Family welfare, New Delhi. NIHFW is act as an apex technical institute as well as a 'think tank' for the promotion of health and family welfare programmes in the country.

48. **Herbal Gram:** Published by American Botanical Council, since 1988, the American Botanical Council (ABC) has been educating consumers, healthcare professionals, researchers, educators, industry and the media on the safe and effective use of herbs and medicinal plants.

49. **Himalayan Journal of Sciences**: Published by the Himalayan Association for the Advancement Journal of Science.

50. **Human Ecology**: An Interdisciplinary Journal publishes papers probing the complex and varied systems of interaction between people and their environment.

51. **Human Organization**: Published by Society for Applied Anthropology. The Society has for its object the promotion of interdisciplinary scientific investigation of the principles controlling the relations of human beings to one another, and the encouragement of the wide application of these principles to practical problems, and shall be known as The Society for Applied Anthropology.

52. **Human Science**: Published by Anthropological Survey of India, Kolkata.

53. **The India Magazine:** A publication of Business India Group.

54. **Indian Anthropologist**: Indian Anthropologist is a journal of an international repute. It is published biannually by Indian Anthropological Association, University of Delhi.

55. **Indian Farming**: Published monthly by the Indian Council of Agricultural Research (ICAR) is an autonomous organization under the Department of Agricultural Research and Education (DARE), Ministry of Agriculture, Government of India. Formerly known as Imperial Council of Agricultural Research, The ICAR has its headquarters at New Delhi.

56. **Indian Forester**: The Indian Forester, a pioneer journal

in the field of Forestry Research established in 1875 has been serving the cause of Scientific Forestry Research since its inception. It is closely associated with the continuous advancement of forestry, and is a storehouse of information for those who want to indulge deep into the progress of forestry in the country.

57. **Indian Indigenous knowledge and development Monitor**: The Indigenous Knowledge and Development Monitor promote the dissemination of local knowledge as a service to the international development community and all scientists who share a professional interest in indigenous knowledge systems and practices. The journal is published three times a year by CIRAN—the Centre for International Research and Advisory Networks, a department of Nuffic (Netherlands organization for international cooperation in higher education) as part of its Indigenous Knowledge Information System.

58. **Indian Journal of Forestry**: M/s Bishen Singh Mahendra Pal Singh

59. **Indian Journal of Fundamental and Applied Life Sciences:** The Indian Journal of Fundamental and Applied Life Sciences (JLS) is an open access online international journal that provides online publication of original research work, review and views in all areas of life sciences from all over the world. Covering current trends in research in life sciences but may be interesting to general readers outside the field.

60. **Indian Journal of Medical Research/ Indian medical Research Memoirs**: Published by the Indian Council of Medical Research (ICMR), New Delhi, the apex body in India for the formulation, coordination and promotion of biomedical research, is one of the oldest medical research bodies in the world.

61. **Indian Journal of Natural Products and Resources**: Published by National Institute of Science Communication and Information Resources, New Delhi. A quarterly journal, is dedicated to the exploration of topics that confront both educators, frontline workers in the fields, entrepreneurs and ultimate users of the value added products and their resources pertaining to both plants and animals. The scope

of the journal is multidisciplinary especially of applied nature.

62. **Indian Journal of Physical Anthropology and Human Genetics**: Published by Serials Publication, New Delhi on behalf of Ethnographic Folk Culture Society, Lucknow.

63. **Indian Journal of Traditional Knowledge**: Published by National Institute of Science Communication and Information Resources, New Delhi.

64. **Indian Journal Orthopedics:** Indian Journal of Orthopaedics journal is official peer-reviewed, open access publication of the Indian Orthopaedic Association (IOA) and is published on Bimonthly basis. IJO is published in first week of January, April, July and October.

65. **Indian Medical Gazette**: Published by connectjournals.com

66. **International Journal of Biology, Pharmacy and allied Science:** International Journal of Biology, Pharmacy and Allied Sciences (IJBPAS) is a peer reviewed, open access online international journal. It is published with an aim to bridge the gap between laboratories and the reader.

67. **International Journal of Crude Drugs Research:** available at http://www.researchgate.net/journal/0167-7314_International_journal_of_crude_drug_research

68. **Journal of Andaman Science Association:** Published by Andaman Science Association, Port Blair

69. **Journal of Anthropological Sociology Bombay:** Published by the Anthropological Society of Bombay.

70. **Journal of Asiatic Society Bengal:** Published by the Asiatic Society Bengal, Kolkata.

71. **Journal of Bombay Natural History Society:** Published by the Bombay Natural History Society, Bombay.

72. **Journal of Economic Botany and Photochemistry:**

73. **Journal of Economic and Taxonomic Botany:** Published by the Society for Economic and Taxonomic Botany (India).

74. **International Journal of Environmental Education and Information:** Devoted to the study of the environment in the broadest sense; provides a multidisciplinary forum for those involved in environmental education and seeks to

promote environmental awareness and education through publishing research, information, experience and knowledge, overviews, and reports.

75. **Journal of Ethnobiology and Ethno-medicine:** *Journal of Ethnobiology and Ethnomedicine* is an open access, peer-reviewed, online journal that aims to promote the exchange of original knowledge and research in any area of ethnobiology and ethnomedicine.

76. **Journal of Ethnopharmacology**: The Journal of Ethnopharmacology is dedicated to the exchange of information and understandings about people's use of plants, fungi, animals, microorganisms and minerals and their biological and pharmacological effects based on the principles established through international conventions and published by the Elsevier Ireland Ltd.

77. **Journal of Herbs, Spices and Medicinal Plants: Published by** Taylor and Francis, Inc., Philadelphia. The Journal of Herbs, Spices and Medicinal Plants is an essential reference filled with recent research and other valuable information associated with herbs, spices, and medicinal plants.

78. **Journal of Himalayan studies and regional development:** Institute of Himalayan Studies and Regional Development. Garhwal University,

79. **Journal of Human Ecology:** Monthly (12 issues 4 Vols. Per year) Published by Kamla Raj Enterprises, New Delhi, full text online available at www.krepublishers.com

80. **Journal of the Indian Anthropological Society:** Published in three issues every year, March, July and November, Published by the Indian Anthropological Society, 27, Jawaharlal Nehru Road, Kolkata.

81. **Journal of Indian Botanical Society:** Published by Indian Botanical Society.

82. **Journal of Medicinal Aromatic plants Science:** Published by Central Institute of Medicinal and Aromatic Plants, Lucknow

83. **Journal of Museum Association of India:** Museums Association of India (MAI) is a registered Society having the

country's well known museologists, historians, archaeologists, conservators, anthropologists, retired/and working curators, research scholars and persons of different fields but interested to be associated with it.

84. **Journal of Non-Timber Forest Products:** Half yearly publication of Bishen Singh Mahendra Pal Singh, Dehradun.

85. **Journal of Pharmaceutical Science and Technology**: Journal of Pharmaceutical Science and Technology, JPST is an international online journal in English that publishes research and review articles in the field of Pharmacy, Pharmaceutical science, science and technology.

86. **Journal of Plants and Nature:**

87. **Journal of Research in Indian Medicine and Homoeopathy:**

88. **Journal of Research in Indian Medicine, Yoga and Homeopathy:**

89. **Journal of Research in Indian Medicine:**

90. **Journal of Science Research Plant Medicine:**

91. **Journal of Social and Economic Studies:**

92. **Journal of Social Research:** Journal of Social Research is an organ of the Department of Anthropology, Ranchi University, Ranchi, published bi-annual.

93. **Journal of Social Science**: Published by Kamala-Raj Enterprises, Delhi. Journal covers, but not limited to, Anthropology, Sociology, Geography, Economics, History, Environmental Studies, Business Administration, Home Science, Public Health, Political Science, Demography, Cultural Studies, Ethnography and Sociolinguistics, along with their interfaces.

94. **Journal of the American Oriental Society:** Published by the American Oriental Society is the oldest learned society in the United States devoted to a particular field of scholarship. The encouragement of basic research in the languages and literatures of Asia has always been central in its tradition. This tradition has come to include such subjects as philology, literary criticism, textual criticism, paleography, epigraphy, linguistics, biography, archaeology, and the history of the intellectual and imaginative aspects

of Oriental civilizations, especially of philosophy, religion, folklore and art.

95. **Journal of the Anthropological Survey of India**: Published by the Anthropological Survey of India, Kolkata.

96. **Journal of University of Poona Science Technology:** A publication of University of Pune, Poona.

97. **Khadigramodyog:** Published by Khadi and Village Industries Commission, India. Khadi and Village Industries Commission.

98. **Kurukshetra**: Published by Publication Division, Ministry of Information and Broad Casting, Government of India.

99. **Lichenologist**: Published on behalf of The British Lichen Society. The Lichenologist is the premier scientific journal devoted exclusively to the study of lichens worldwide.

100. **Madhya Bharati**: A research journal of Dr. Hari Singh Gour Central University, Sagar (M.P.)

101. **Man and Environment**: Published bi-annual by the Indian Society for Prehistoric and Quaternary Studies, Department of Archaeology, Deccan College, Pune.

102. **Man in India:** A Quarterly Journal Founded in 1921 by Sarat Chandra Roy, Published by the Serial Publications, New Delhi, India.

103. **Man and Life**: Published by the Institute of Social Research and Applied Anthropology, Bidisa (West Bengal).

104. **Manipur University Museum Bulletin**: Published by Manipur University Museum. It is a full – fledged multi purpose department catering to the needs and requirements of the students and Research Scholars mainly in the fields of Art and Culture, Archaeology, History, Natural History etc.

105. **Mountain Research Development**: Mountain Research and Development fosters sustainable development in mountains by supporting peer-reviewed interdisciplinary, disciplinary, and transdisciplinary research on mountains, developing scientific capacity, capitalizing on development experiences, promoting policy dialogue, and strengthening networks within the mountain community.

106. **Natural Resources Journal**: The Natural Resources

Journal (NRJ) is published by the University of New Mexico School of Law and is an international, interdisciplinary forum devoted to the study of natural and environmental resources.

107. **Oriental Anthropologist**: The Official organ of The Oriental Institute of Cultural and Social Research, Allahabad (India). The Oriental Anthropologist is a peer reviewed IBSS listed International Journal that Publishes original articles of theoretical, empirical, and applied nature, book reviews, news items, reports of meetings and professional announcements, and debates on current issues in the field of social science in general and anthropology in particular.

108. **Pahar:** Published by the Peoples Association for Hill Area Research, Nainital, Uttaranchal, India.

109. **Pharmaceutical Biology:** Published by Informa Healthcare, London.

110. **Puratattva (Bulletin of the Indian Archaeological Society)**: Indian Archaeological Society is a registered (under Indian Society of Registration Act 1860) educational and charitable Institution.

111. **Quarterly Journal of Crude Drug Research:**

112. **Quarterly Journal of Drug Research:**

113. **Quarterly Journal of the Mythic Society**: Published by The Mythic Society, Bangalore

114. **Sachitra Ayurveda:** Published by the Shri Vaidyanath Ayurveda Bhavan, Patna.

115. **Science and Environment:**

116. **Science and Culture**: The Indian Science News Association was established in 1935 with the initiative of Professor Meghnad Saha and Acharya P.C. Ray with an objective to disseminate science news as well as the reflection of the community of Indian scientists and thinkers for public understanding of science and culture together. To meet this goal the Association has been publishing a journal Science and Culture from its inception.

117. **Social Action**: Social Action has been published continuously since 1951 by the Indian Social Institute. This Journal has been capturing the social dimension of independent India. It is now published by the Social Action

Trust. The Journal attempts to reach activists in the field with committed intellectual and theoretical concerns, as well as intellectuals and academics seriously committed to action in the field.

118. **Social Science Medicine:** Provides an international and interdisciplinary forum for the dissemination of social science research on health.

119. **South Asian Anthropologist**: Published by Serials Publications, South Asian Anthropologist, a biannual peer reviewed journal (March-September), publishes original articles in the field of anthropology, sociology, demography, human biology, environmental studies, medical anthropology, tribal and rural economy, and development studies, etc.

120. **South Indian Folklorist:** Published by Folklore Resources and Research Centre, St. Xavier's College (Autonomous) Tirunelveli, Tamil Nadu.

121. **Soviet Anthropology and Archaeology**: Published by International Arts and Sciences Press, New York.

122. **Studies on Ethno-medicine**: published by Kamla-Raj Enterprises, Delhi. Study on ethno-medicine is a peer reviewed internationally circulated journal. It publishes theoretical articles and timely reviews, and brief communications in the interdisciplinary field of Ethno-medicine.

123. **Swasth Hind:** Central Health Education Bureau (Directorate General of Health Services) India.

124. **The Hindu**: The Hindu, started in 1878 as a weekly, became a daily in 1889 and from then on has been steadily growing to the circulation of 14,66,304 copies (ABC: July-December 2009) and a readership of about 4.06 million.

125. **The Journal of Family Practice**: The Journal of Family Practice is a source of original research and evidence-based medical information for practicing family physicians, family medicine researchers, and other primary care clinicians.

126. **The Journal of Research and Education in Indian Medicine**: The Journal of Research and education in Indian Medicine (JREIM) is a quarterly peer-reviewed international

journal. JREIM has been established and launched in 1982 by a group of dedicated academicians and researchers of Ayurveda and allied disciplines under the dynamic leadership of Padamshree Prof. K. N. Udupa, the than Director, Institute of Medical Sciences, Banaras Hindu University, Varanasi (India).

127. **Tribal Health Bulletin**: Regional Medical Research Centre for Tribals Jabalpur, (MP).

128. **Tribal Research Bulletin, Maharashtra**: Published by Tribal Research & Training Institute, Pune.

129. **Vanyajati:** A Quarterly Journal in English and Hindi, Published by the Bhartiya Adimjati Sevak Sangh, New link road, Jhadewala, New Delhi, India. Vegetos.

130. **World Health Forum:** Published by the WHO.

131. **Yojana**: Published by Publication Division, Ministry of Information and Broadcasting, Govt. of India. Yojana is a monthly devoted to socio-economic issues and started its publication in 1957 with Mr. Khuswant Singh as its Chief Editor. The magazine is now published in 13 languages viz. English, Hindi, Urdu, Punjabi, Marathi, Gujarati, Bengali, Assamese, Telugu, Tamil, Kannada, Malayalam and Oriya.

Introduction

INTANGIBLE CULTURAL HERITAGE OF INDIA: AN OVERVIEW

Kamal K. Misra

The saga of human history and civilization is replete with examples that testify the fact that unprecedented technological sophistication and unswerving process of globalization of our times have not come without a price. They have a leveling effect on human culture, thus alarmingly shrinking the cultural diversity. The eco-specific cultural patterns and amazingly varied languages are now rushing towards greater uniformity, thus losing individual identities of peoples and their cultures. There is, therefore, a threat to the cultural heritage of the humankind.

But what is cultural heritage? The International Council on Monuments and Sites (ICOMOS) has defined that "Cultural Heritage is an expression of the ways of living developed by a community and passed on from generation to generation, including customs, practices, places, objects, artistic expressions and values." (2002). The process of globalization has not only reduced distance considerably, but also brought information and commodities much closer to the people. With the increase in buying power and easy availability of information and commodities, preferences are more towards those which look glamorous and fascinating. Examples of this trend are many; the songs that marked beginning of a season, celebration of birth or marriage, or a mourning in rural and tribal India are now replaced by cinema songs. This is how the distinctiveness of identity is in peril and cultural heritage is threatened.

Cultural Heritage is a much wider concept. John Feather (2006) has aptly said that the driving force behind all definitions of cultural heritage is a human creation intended to inform. It informs all that is created and maintained by the people as a part of their distinct culture. It could be built environments, such as buildings, townscapes and archaeological remains; natural environments, such as rural landscapes; artifacts, such as manuscripts, documents, material objects or pictures; or the ideas and the skills behind all the above mentioned creations and innovations. Therefore, cultural heritage could be either tangible or intangible. In the UNESCO document it is stated that "Cultural heritage is not limited to material manifestations, such as monuments and objects that have been preserved over time. This notion also encompasses living expressions and the traditions that countless groups and communities worldwide have inherited from their ancestors and transmit to their descendants, in most cases orally." While the former is the tangible aspects of the cultural heritage that underlines the visible traces from human antiquity to the recent times, the latter connotes the intangible or "living heritage" representing the value systems, beliefs, traditions and lifestyles of the people that are mostly transmitted orally.

According to the Donald Horne Institute of Cultural Heritage at the University of Canberra, cultural heritage and its recognition and preservation were not taken seriously till recent times. As a field of scholarship, cultural heritage emerged over the past forty or fifty years when universities in the West diversified beyond the traditional disciplines into new fields of cross-disciplinary or multi-disciplinary enquiry. Simultaneously, collections in museums, archives, libraries and galleries became a topic of study in their own right, so too did national parks, sacred places, historic buildings and entire landscapes. When the National Trusts, National Parks Associations and activist citizens groups started propagating the value of cultural heritages and started protecting them, popular awareness about cultural heritage gained momentum. The UNESCO contributed to the recognition and protection of cultural heritages of nations in a big way. Many governments and non-government agencies also joined their hands in this process. Popular consciousness got heightened with the rapid pace of globalization, mono-culturalism and ruthless destruction of priceless cultural heritages all over the world.

India's cultural heritage is rich and diverse due to its civilizational past. It is represented by thousands of monuments, temples and other works of art, such as paintings, sculptures and handicrafts found across the length and breadth of this country. Besides these tangible heritages are the less visible forms of cultural heritages, pertaining to oral traditions, aesthetic and religious beliefs, rituals and festivals, arts, music, folk traditions, dances, theatre forms, performing arts and narrative styles of storytelling. They are the insignia of the rich and diverse, multi-cultural, multi–linguistic cultural heritage of India. These are also called traditional expressions and include oral literature, music, dance, games, mythology, rituals, costumes and crafts. Sometimes the cultural spaces, such as sites for story-telling, rituals and festivals, market places, where traditional cultural activities take place, are also included under the intangible cultural heritage.

Now we might question the relevance of understanding and protecting cultural heritage of the people and nations, particularly the intangible cultural heritage. The UNESCO document states that "While fragile, intangible cultural heritage is an important factor in maintaining cultural diversity in the face of growing globalization. An understanding of the intangible cultural heritage of different communities helps with intercultural dialogue, and encourages mutual respect for other ways of life. The importance of intangible cultural heritage is not the cultural manifestation itself but rather the wealth of knowledge and skills that is transmitted through it from one generation to the next. The social and economic value of this transmission of knowledge is relevant for minority groups and for mainstream social groups within a State, and is as important for developing States as for developed ones."

The UNESCO document suggests the following features of intangible cultural heritage or the living heritage:

(1) It is traditional, contemporary and living at the same time. This means that although inherited cultural traditions from the past are very important intangible heritages, it does not preclude the contemporary rural and urban cultural practices undertaken by diverse groups and communities as their heritage.

(2) It is inclusive or a shared expression that is similar to those practiced by many different groups and communities. Acculturation and spatial mobility are the hallmarks of human civilization. As a result, it is likely that similar practices may be observed in different villages, cities, and even in different corners of the world when the diasporic communities continue to practice them to express their origin and identity. These are all intangible cultural heritages, although they might have changed a bit due to their adaptation to the local environments. In any case they give a sense of identity and continuity, providing a link from our past, through the present, and into our future. It fosters social cohesion through the process of sharing of heritages.

(3) Intangible cultural heritage represents peoples and communities and depends upon those whose knowledge of traditions, skills and customs are transmitted to the rest of the community from one generation to the other or from one to other communities.

(4) Intangible cultural heritages have to be recognized as such by the groups, communities or individuals who create, maintain and transmit them. Without their recognition, none can decide them as heritages on their behalf.

Given the scope and spread of intangible cultural heritage or living heritage of India, there could be a huge list that includes many traditions, practices and customs as outlined earlier. For example, stories, family events, community gatherings, languages and dialects, songs, knowledge of natural and cultural spaces, healing traditions, food and beverages, recreation activities, beliefs and cultural practices, skills, performing arts, etc., which we inherit generationally and share between groups and communities. The Janapada Sampada Division of the Indira Gandhi National Centre of Art (IGNCA) has prepared an inventory of 30 elements (sic. items) under intangible cultural heritage of India. The list includes Buddhist chanting of Ladakh, Chaar Bayt, Dashavatar, the festival of Salhesh, Hingan paintings, Kalbelia dance and songs, and many more (http://www.ignca.nic.in/ich_ inventory.htm).

Eastern India's Chhau dance, Kalbelia folk songs and dances of Rajasthan, and Mudiyettu ritual theater and dance drama of Kerala have already found place in the UNESCO representative list of intangible cultural heritage of humanity. The Indira Gandhi Rashtriya Manav Sangrahalaya had earlier made an attempt to include the Nacha folk theater of Chhatisgarh and the Vaishnav Satriya tradition of Majuli islands in Assam under the UNESCO list of intangible cultural heritages of India.

India undoubtedly is a rich repository of intangible cultural heritages due to its cultural diversity. But many of these heritages have already disappeared or are endangered due to the relentless sway of globalization and mono-culturalism. The need of the hour, therefore, is to document whatever little still exists and protect them for the posterity. The World Intellectual Property Organization (WIPO) based in Geneva has been making all out efforts to prepare international legal instruments for the protection of genetic resources, traditional knowledge and traditional cultural expressions including folklore, so that they could be protected from unethical piracy and those who innovate, practice and protect them could be benefited.

Realizing the importance of intangible cultural heritages of India and their documentation, Indira Gandhi Rashtriya Manav Sangrahalaya has undertaken the task of preparing selective bibliographies on various aspects of intangible cultural heritages to facilitate scholars and researchers in their pursuit of knowledge. It is proposed to be a multi-volume exercise due to enormous literature available on the subject. While the Volume I intends to cover fairs, festivals, customs, beliefs, ceremonies, rites, rituals, manners and traditions, the Volume II incorporates ethno-medical practices in India. Subsequent volumes on other aspects of intangible cultural heritage of India would follow these volumes soon. If these volumes indeed help and inspire scholars in the field of intangible cultural heritage, our efforts would be encouraging and productive.

References

Bhela, Anita (2001) Preserving India's Intangible Cultural Heritage: Issues and Challenges, International Journal of the Humanities, 8 (5), 207-214.

Feather, John (2006) Managing the Documentary Heritage: Issues from the Present and Future. In, Gorman, G.E. and Sydney

J. Shep (eds.) Preservation Management for Libraries, Archives and Museums, 1-18, London: Facet.

http://www.unesco.org/culture/ich/doc/src/01851-EN.pdf.

http://www.canberra.edu.au/centres/donald-horne/cultural-heritage/what-is.

http://www.ignca.nic.in/ich_inventory.htm.

Bibliography

1. Aacharya, Deepak and Shrivastava, Anshu "Indigenous herbal medicines: Tribal formulations and traditional herbal practices". Jaipur, Avishkar Publishers Distributors, 2008.
2. Abdin, M. Z. and Abrol, Y. P. "Traditional systems of medicine". Alpha Science International Ltd./Narosa Publishing House, 2006, p. 567.
3. Abraham, Leena "Medicine as culture: Indigenous medicine in cosmopolitan Mumbai". *Economic and Political Weekly*, Vol. 44, No 16, 2009, pp. 68-75.
4. Abraham, Rony "Relax, revive and rejuvenate". *Discover India*, Vol. 13, No. 8, 2000, pp. 48-49.
5. Abraham, S. Annie "Traditional medicines for sustainable health care and community development". *Yojana,* Vol. 55, March 2011, pp. 54-58.
6. Abraham, Z. "Ethnobotany of the Todas, the Kotas and the Irulas of the Nilgiris". In Glimpses of Indian ethnobotany, edited by S. K. Jain, New Delhi, Oxford & IBH Publishing Co., pp. 308-320.
7. Acharya, Sabita "Health, disease and indigenous health are system among the Munda: A primitive tribe of Orissa". In Traditional knowledge in contemporary societies: Challenges and apportunities, edited by Kamal K. Misra, IGRMS, Bhopal & Pratibha Prakashan, Delhi, 2007, pp. 258-273.
8. Acharyya, B. K. and Sharma, H. K. "Folklore medicinal plants of Mahmora area, Sivasagar district, Assam". *Indian Journal of Traditional Knowledge,* Vol. 3, No. 4, 2004, pp. 365-372.
9. Ackerknecht, E. H. "On the collection of data concerning

primitive medicine". *American Anthropologist*, Vol. 47, 1945, pp. 427-432.

10. Ackerknecht, E. H. "Problems of primitive medicine". *Bulletin of the History of Medicine*, Vol. 11, 1942, pp. 503-21.
11. Ackernecht, E. H. "Natural disease and rational treatment primitive medicine". *Bulletin of the History of Medicine*, Vol. 19, No. 5, 1946, pp. 467-497.
12. Agarwal, V. S. and Saha, S. "Unreported medicinal plants of India". *Journal of Andhra Pradesh Academic Science*, Vol. 2, 1968, pp. 21-23.
13. Aggarwal, Hemla and Kotwal, Nidhi "Foods used as ethno-medicine in Jammu". *Studies in Ethno-medicine*, Vol. 3, No. 1, 2009, pp. 65-68.
14. Agrawal, Pramod, S. Deshmukh, Asif Ali, S. Patil, C. S. Magdum, S. K. Mohite and T. D. Nandgude "Wild flowers as medicines". *International Journal of Green Pharmacy*, Vol. 1, No. 1, 2007, pp. 12-13.
15. Agrawal, V. S. "Ancient Indian folk cults", Varansi, 1970.
16. Agrawal, V. S. "Roots of Indian plants as source for medicines". *Indian Museum Bulletin*, Vol. 4, No. 2, 1969, pp. 81-101.
17. Ahluwalia, Aneeta "Sociology of medicine in India: An approach", *Economic and Political Weekly*, Vol. 2, No. 22, 1967, pp. 1007-1012.
18. Ahluwalia, K. S. "Medicinal plants of Har-Ki-Dun, Toons division, U.P.". *Nagarjun,* Vol. 8, 1965, pp. 135-139.
19. Ahmad, J. and Chaghtai, S. A. "A study of tree flora of Bhopal with special reference to their medicinal values". *Bulletin of Medicinal and Ethnobotany Research*, Vol. 3, No. 1, 1982, pp. 114-152.
20. Ahmed, J. "Medicinal uses of dry and common fruits used in indigenous system of medicine- part I". *Nagarjun*, Vol. 21, No. 12, 1978, pp. 25-29.
21. Ahuja, P. S. "Current status of propagation of medicinal plants in Indian Himalaya". In Himalayan medicinal plants: Potential and prospects edited by S. S. Samant, U. Dhar and L. M. S. Palni, Gyanodaya Prakasan, Nainital, 2001, pp. 207-231.

22. Aiman, R. "Indigenous anti-diabetic substance of plant origin". *Indian Journal of Pharmacology*, Vol. 23, 1961, pp. 115.

23. Aiyyapan, A. A. "Primitive medicine at a Malabar temple". *Indian Journal of Historical Medicine*, Vol. 2, 1957, pp. 37-42.

24. Akerele, O. "Role of traditional medicine in health-care delivery system". Paper presented at the first international seminar on Unani medicine, New Delhi, Feb. 13-15, 1987.

25. Akhtar, Rais (ed.) "Disease ecology and health: readings in medical geography". Jaipur, Rawat Publications, 1990, p. 314.

26. Alagesaboopathi, C. "Ethnomedicinal plants and their utilization by villagers in Kumaragiri Hills of Salem district of Tamil Nadu, India". *African Journal of Traditional, Complementary and Alternative Medicine*, Vol. 6, No. 3, 2009, pp. 222-227.

27. Alagesaboopathi, C., Dwarakan, P. and Balu, S. "Plants used as medicine by tribals of Shevaroy Hills, Tamil Nadu". In Ethnobotany and medicinal plant of Indian subcontinent, edited by J. K. Maheshwari, Saujanya Books, Jodhpur, 2003, p. 672.

28. Alagesaboopathi, C., Dwarakan, P. and Ramachandran, V. S. "Andrographis paniculata Nees in tribal medicine of Tamil Nadu". *Ancient Science of Life*, Vol. 19, No. 1&2, 1999, pp. 28-30.

29. Alavi, Seema "Islam and healing-loss and recovery of an Indo-muslim medical tradition 1600-1900". Permanent Black, Ranikhet, 2008, p. 384.

30. Alcorn, Janis B. "Ethnobotanical knowledge systems: A resources for meeting rural development goals". In indigenous knowledge systems: the cultural dimension of development, edited by D. M. Warren, David Brokensha and L. Jan Slikkerveer, London, Kegan Paul International, 1992.

31. Ali, Almas "Indigenous health practices among tribals: relationship with prevalent diseases". In Tribal health in India, edited by Salil Basu, Delhi: Manak Publications, 1994, pp. 130-150.

32. Ali, Almas, "Tribal health research: Issues and challenges". Paper presented at the national workshop on tribal health and medicine in forest environment". Dept. of KIRTADS, Kozhikode, Kerala, 1987.

33. Ali, Md. Arif "Studies on folk medicine in tribal India: A bibliography for the intrested scholars". *Folklore*, Vol. 32, No. 9, 1991, pp. 149-153; 161.

34. Ali, Momin "Role of indigenous medicine in primary health-care". Paper present at the 1st International Seminar on Unani Medicine, New Delhi, Feb. 13-15, 1987.

35. Aliya, S. D. "Use of some Indian plants in folkmedicines of Nepal". *Ethnobotany*, Vol. 17, No. 1&2, 2005, pp. 202-204.

36. Alphen, Jan Van and Aris, Anthony "Oriental medicine: an illustrated guide to Asian art of healing". Serindia Publications Inc., 1995, p. 271.

37. Alves, Romulo Romeu da Nobrega, Vieisra, Washington Luiz da Silva and Santana, Gindomar Gomes "Reptiles used in traditional folk medicine: conservation implications". *Biodiversity and Conservation*, Vol. 17, No. 8, 2008, pp. 2037-2049.

38. Ambasta, S.P. "The useful plants of India". Publication and Information Directorate, CSIR, New Delhi, 1986.

39. Aminuddin and Girach, R.D. "Observations on Ethnobotany of the Bhunjia : A tribe of Sonabera Plateau". *Ethnobotany*, Vol. 5, No. 1 & 2, 1993, pp. 83-86.

40. Aminuddin, and Girach, G. D. "Ethnobotanical studies on Bondo tribe of district Koraput (Orissa), India". *Ethnobotany*, Vol. 3, 1991, pp. 15-19.

41. Aminudin "Search for anti-malarial drugs in the tribal pockets of Orissa", Paper present at the 1st seminar on Unani medicine, New Delhi, Feb. 13-15, 1987.

42. Anand, R. M. and others "A survey of medicinal plants in Kollimalai hill tracts, Tamil Nadu". *Indian Journal of Natural Products and Resources*, Vol. 5, No. 2, 2006, pp. 139-143.

43. Anderson, E. "Plants, man and life". University of California Press, Berkeley, 1967.

44. Angami, A., Gajurel, P. R. and Rethy, P. "Status and

potential of wild edible plants of Arunachal Pradesh". *Indian Journal of Traditional Knowledge,* Vol. 5, No. 4, 2006, pp. 541-550.

45. Anil Kumar and Misra, K.K. "Ethno-medicinal practices and ethnic healers among the Konda Reddi of Andhra Pradesh". In Reproductive and Child Health: Social cultural dimensions, edited by R.N. Pati, New Delhi, Ashish, 2003, pp. 1-20.

46. Anil, K.M. "Ethno-hermeneutics: A theory on culture to elicit meaning", *South Indian Folklorist*, Vol. 8, 2005, pp. 111-120.

47. Anis, M. and Iqbal, A. "Antipyretic utility of some Indian plants in traditional medicine". *Fitoterapia*, Vol. 57, No. 1, 1986, pp. 52-55.

48. Annon. "Contant therapy practised by Mundas of Chotanagpur: (Bihar)" *Ethnobotany,* Vol. 8, No. 1&2, 1996, pp. 36-39.

49. Annon. "Health and disease in tribal societies". Ciba Foundation Symposium, Vol. 49, Amesterdam, Elsevier Excerpta Medica, 1977.

50. Annon. "Indigenous medicine losing favour". *The Times of India*, September 9, 2011.

51. Annon. "Nature's healing arts: From folk medicine to modern drugs", *National Geographic Society*, Washington D.C. 1977.

52. Annon. "Need for action research for health development among tribal communities of India". *South Asian Anthropologist,* Vol. 17, No. 2, 1996, pp. 73-80.

53. Annon. "Ramban ausadhi gaumootra". *Ojaswani,* March, 2006, pp. 27. [Hindi]

54. Annon. "Swasthvardhak ausadhiy vanaspatiyon se swayam hi ausadhiya banane ki vidhiyan". Koyambatoor, Lok Swasthya Prampara Sambardhan Samiti, 1995, p. 62. [Hindi]

55. Annon. "Thannane Thawe: Tribal medicine issue". Bangalore, Kaavya, 1997, p. 178. [Tamil]

56. Annon. "The politics of being 'Indigenous'". In Indigeneity

in India, edited by Bengt G. Karlsson and T.B. Subba, Kegan Paul Limited London, 2006, pp. 33-46.

57. Annon. "Traditional medicine- views from the South -East Asia region". *WHO Chronicle*, Vol. 31, No. 2, 1974, pp. 47-52.

58. Annon. "Visha chikitsa: a manual on poisonous bites and its management in traditional medicine". Coimbatore, LSPSS, p. 29.

59. Ansari, A. A. and Ghana Nand "Some medicinal plants of Pauri Garhwal". *Himalayan Chemical Pharmacy Bulletin*, Vol. 2, 1985, pp. 42-44.

60. Anuradha, R. V. "Mainstreaming indigenous knowledge: developing 'Jeevani'". *Economic and Political weekly*, Vol. 33, No. 26, 1998, pp.1615-1619.

61. Apparanantham, T. and Chelladurai, V. "Glimpses of folk medicines of Dharampuri forest division, Tamil Nadu". *Ancient Science of Life*, Vol. 5, 1986, pp. 182-185.

62. Arber, A. "Herbals, their origin and evolution". Cambridge, Cambridge University Press, 1938.

63. Archer, M. "The folktalk in Santal society". *Man in India*, Vol. 24, 1944, pp. 224-32.

64. Archer, M. "The Santhal treatment of wichcraft". *Man in India,* Vol. 27, 1987, p. 103.

65. Arenas, P. and Azorero, R. M. "Plants of commaon use in paraguayan folk medicine for regulating fertility". *Economic Botany*, Vol. 31, 1977, pp. 298-301.

66. Arenas, P. and Azorero, R. M. "Plants used as means of abortion, contraception, sterlization and fecundation by Praguayan indigenous people". *Economic Botany*, Vol. 31, 1977, pp. 302-306.

67. Arif Hasan, K. "The cultural frontier of health in village India: Case study of a North Indian Village". Manaktalas, Bombay, 1967.

68. Arinathan, V. and Moihan, V. R. "Wild edibles used by Palliyars of the Western Ghats, Tamil Nadu". *Indian Journal of Traditional Knowledge,* Vol. 6, No. 1, 2007, pp. 163-168.

69. Arnold, David (ed.) "Imperial medicine and indigenous societies". Delhi, Oxford University press. 1989, p. 231.

70. Arora, Kavita "Sustainable management of tropical forest through indigenous knowledge: A case study of Shompens of great Nicobar Island". *Indian Journal of Traditional Knowledge,* Vol. 9, No. 3, 2009, pp. 551-561.

71. Arora, R. K. "Native food plants of the tribals of Bastar (Madhya Pradesh) India". In Glimpses of Indian Ethnobotany, edited by S.K. Jain, Oxford University Press and IBH, New Delhi, 1981, pp. 91-106.

72. Arya, K. R. and Agarwal, S. C. "Folk therapy for eczema, bone fracture, boils, sores and gingivitis in Taragtal province of Uttaranchal". *Indian Journal of Traditional Knowledge,* Vol. 7, No. 3, 2008, pp. 443-445.

73. Arya, K. R. and Agarwal, S. C. "Survey of herbal folk remedy for piles". *Ethnobotany*, Vol. 13, No. 1-2, 2001, pp. 142-145.

74. Arya, K.R., Pande, P.C. and Ved Prakash, "Ethnobotanical study on tribal areas of Almora district- II". *Ethnobotany,* Vol. 11, No. 1&2, 1999, pp. 100-104.

75. Arya, P. "Mahagatha vrikshon ki". Radhakrishan Prakashan, New Delhi, 1997. [Hindi]

76. Arya, S.P. "Plant lore of West Uttar Pradesh". *Folklore,* Vol. 6, 1965, pp. 114-146,

77. Ashaletha, S. and Immanuel, Sheela "Scope of ethnofisheries and sustainable marine fisheries management in India". *Indian Journal of Traditional Knowledge,* Vol. 7, No. 2, 2009, pp. 226-232.

78. Aswal, B.S. "Conservation of ethnomedicinal plants diversity of Garhwal Himalayain India". In Ethnobiology of Human Welfare edited by S. K. Jain, Deep Publications, New Delhi. 1996, pp. 133-135.

79. Aswal, B.S. "Less known medicinal uses of three plants from Kumaun Himalaya (India)". *Indian Journal of Forestry*, Vol. 15, No. 1, 1992, pp. 76-77.

80. Aswal, B.S. and Goel, A.K. "Less-known medicinal uses of three plants from Western Himalaya (India)". *Economic Botany*, Vol. 43, 1989, pp. 419-420.

81. Atique, A. "Use of anona squamosa and piper nigrum against diabetes". *Fitoterapia*, Vol. 56, No. 3, 1985, pp. 190-192.

82. Atique, A. M., Iqbal, M. and Ghouse, A. K. M. "Folk medicinal uses of ficus bengalensis Linn. and punica granatum linn in Northern Uttar Pradesh". *Bulletin of Medico-ethnobotanical Rresearch*, Vol. 6, 1985, pp. 42-46.

83. Atre, Subhash "Chhattisgarh lok jeevan me vanaspati evam ausadhi". *Chaumasa*, Vol. 18, No. 57, 2002, pp. 109-111. [Hindi]

84. Audichya, K.C., Billore, K. V., Joseph, T. H. and Chaturvedi, D. D. "Role of indigenous folk remedies for certain acute illness in primary health care". *Nagarjun*, Vol. 26, No. 9, 1983, pp. 199-201.

85. Augustine, Jomy and Sivadasan, M. "Ethnomedicinal plants of Periyar Tiger Reserve, Kerala, India". *Ethnobotany*, Vol. 16, No. 1&2, 2004, pp. 142-145.

86. Awasthi, A. K. "Folklore medico-botany of the aboriginal inhabitants of Andaman and Nicobar Islands". *Journal of Andaman Science Association*, Vol. 3, No. 2, 1987, pp. 80-87.

87. Awasthi, A. K. and Goel, Anil K. "Ethnobotanical studies on the tribe Onge from little Andaman island". In Ethnobotany and medicinal plant of Indian subcontinent, edited by J. K. Maheshwari, Saujanya Books, Jodhpur, 2003, p. 672.

88. Ayensu, E. S. "Endengered plants used in traditional medicine". In Traditional medicine and health care coverage edited by R. H. Bannermann and others, Geneva, World Health Organization, 1983.

89. Ayyanar, M. and Ignacimuthu, S. "Traditional knowledge of Kani tribals in Kouthalai of Tirunelveli hills, Tamil Nadu, India". *Journal of Ethnopharmacology*, Vol. 102, 2005, pp. 246-255.

90. Babbar, O. P. et al. "Occurrence of interferon like anti-viral and anti-tumour factors in extracts of some indigenous plants". *Indian Journal of of Experimental Biology*, Vol. 17, 1979, pp. 451-454.

91. Babu, M. Hari, Prasanthi, S. and Reddi, T. V. V. Seetharami

"Plant based native therapy for piles in Visakhapatnam district of Andhra Pradesh". *Ethnobotany,* Vol. 22, No. 1-2, 2010, pp. 114-117.

92. Bachchan Kumar "Bhils: an ethno-historic analysis". Delhi, Sharada Publishing House, 1997, p. 244.

93. Badami, Shrishailappa and Rai, Sujay "In-vitro antioxidant properties of Indian traditonal paan and its ingredients". *Indian Journal of Traditional Knbowledge*, Vol. 3, No. 2, 2004, pp. 187-191.

94. Badami, Shrishailappa Moorkoth, Sudheer B., Suresh "Caesalpinia sappan – A medicinal and dye yield plant". *Indian Journal of Natural Products and Resources,* Vol. 3, No. 2, 2004, pp. 75-82.

95. Badgujar, S.B. and Patil, M.B. "Ethnomedicines for jaundice used in tribal areas of North Maharashtra". *Natural Product Radiance,* Vol. 7, No. 1, 2008, pp.79-81.

96. Badhe, P.D. and Sharma, B.N. "Ethno-medical methods of Korku tribes of West Melghaṭ". *Bulletin of Medico-Ethnobotanical Research*, Vol. 3, No. 2-4, 1982, pp. 162-172.

97. Badhwar, R.L. "The role of minor forests products for the betterment of tribal and backward classs people". *Indian Forestry*, Vol. 81, 1955, pp. 717-720.

98. Badola H. K., Aitken, S. "The Himalayas of India: A treasury of medicinal plants under siege". *Biodiversity*, Vol. 4, 2003, pp. 3-13.

99. Badoni, A. K. "An ethnobotanical study of Pinswari community: A preliminary survey". *Bulletin of the Botanical Survey of India*, Vol. 32, 1990, pp. 103-115.

100. Badoni, A. K. "Ethnobotany of hill tribes of Uttarkashi, plants used in rituals and psychomedicinal practices". *Journal of Himalayan Studies and regional Development*, Vol. 11-12, 1987-88, pp. 103-115.

101. Badoni, A. K. "Garhwal Himalaya me jaivik vividhata evam satat vikas hetu jari booti udhyog". Society of Himalayan Environmental and Development, Vikasnagar, Dehradun, 1995. [Hindi]

102. Badoni, A. K. "Remarks on the high altitudinal medicinal

plants of Garhwal Himalaya". *Journal of Himalayan Studies & Regional Development*, Vol. 13-14, 1989-90, pp. 37-45.

103. Badoni, A. K. "Some aspects of the ethnobotany of the hill tribes of Uttarkashi district". Proceedings of Indian Botanical Conference, Vol. 65, 1986, pp. 57-58.

104. Badoni, Arun and Badoni, Kiran "Ethnobotanical heritage". In Garhwal Himalaya: Nature, Culture and Society edited by O. P. Kandari and O. P. Gusain, Transmedia, Media House, Srinagar, Garhwal, 2001, pp. 127-147.

105. Bagchi, Niloy Kumar and Ghosh, G. C. "Indigenous health practices among Bhumij of Puruliya district of West Bengal". *Human Science*, Vol. 36, No. 2, 1987, pp. 142-149.

106. Bahulkar, S.S. "Medical ritual in the Atharvaveda tradition". Pune, Tilak Maharashtra Vidyapeeth, Shri Balmukund Sanskrit Mahavidyalaya Research Series No. 8, 1994.

107. Baishya, C.L. and Majumdar, R. "Folklore claims from the Brahmaputra Valley, Assam". *Ethnomedicine,* Vol. 6, 1980, pp. 139-145.

108. Bajpayee, Kaptain K. and Shukla, Ajay K. "Studies on some folk-medicinal plants used in various skin diseases in Hardoi district (U.P.)". *Vanyajati,* Vol. 58, No. 2, 2010, pp. 3-8.

109. Bajpayee, Kaptain Kishor and Dixit, Gopal "Ethnobotanical studies on food-stuffs of tribals of Tarai region, Uttar Pradesh". In Ethnobotany and medicinal plants of Indian Sub-continent, edited by J. K. Maheshwari, Jodhpur, India Scientific Publishers, 2000.

110. Baker, H. G. "Plants and civilization". 2nd edition, Wadsworth Publishing Company, Belmont California, 1970.

111. Bakshi, D. N. "Lexicon of medicinal plants in India (Vol. 1.) "Calcutta, Naya Prokash, 1999. p. 552.

112. Bala, Poonam "Imperialism and medicine in Bengal: A socio-historical perspective". New Delhi, Sage, 1991, p. 174.

113. Balapure, K.M., Maheshwari, J.K. and Tandan, R. K. "Plants of Ramayana". *Ancient Science of life*, Vol. 7, No. 2, 1987, pp. 76-84.

114. Balaramiah, V. "The greatness of siddha medicine". Madras, Aruljothi Publishers, 1973.

115. Balasubramaniam, A. V. "People's knowledge in health care". In Reading Material in Local Health Traditions, edited by TSM, Foundation for Revitalization of Local Health Traditions, Bangalore, FRLHT, 2000, pp.17-26.

116. Balasubramanian, A. V. "Local health traditions: an introduction". Madras, Lok Swasthya Parampara Samvardhan Samithi, 1989, p.95.

117. Balasubramanian, D. "Resurrecting traditional medicine". Science Reporter, Vol. 37, No. 4, 2000, pp. 9-19.

118. Balasubramanian, P. and Prasad, S. Narendra "Medicinal plants among the Irulas of Attappady and Boluvampatti forests in the Nilgiri Biosphere Reserve". In Ethnobotany and medicinal plants of Indian Sub-continent, edited by J. K. Maheshwari, Jodhpur, India Scientific Publishers, 2000.

119. Balkrishna, Gowda and others "Conservation and utilization of medicinal plants by Kudibi tribals in Western Ghats-Karnataka". In Indigenous medicinal plants: including microbes and fungi edited by Purshotam Kaushik, Today and tomorrow's printers and Publishers, New Delhi, 1988, pp. 167-170.

120. Ballabh, Basant and Chaurasia, O. P. "Ethnobotanical studies on Boto tribe in Ladakh". *Ethnobotany*, Vol. 18, No. 1-2, 2006, pp. 87- 95.

121. Ballabh, Basant and Chaurasia, O. P. "Medicinal plants of cold desert Ladakh used in the treatment of stomach disorders". *Indian Journal of Traditional Knowledge,* Vol. 8, No. 2, 2009, pp. 185-190.

122. Balu, S., Alagesaboopathi, C. and Madhavan, S. "Botanical remedies for diabetes from the Cauvery delta of Tamil Nadu". In Ethnobotany and medicinal plant of Indian subcontinent, edited by J. K. Maheshwari, Saujanya Books, Jodhpur, 2003, p. 672.

123. Bandhopadhyay, S. and Mukherjee, Shobhan Kr. "Ethnoveterinary medicine from Koch Bihar district, West Bengal". *Indian Journal of Traditional Knowledge,* Vol. 4, No. 4, 2005, pp. 456-461.

124. Bandyopadhyay, Mousumi "Indigenous approach to infantile mortality and delivery". In History of medicine in India: The medical encounter, edited by Chittabrata Palit and Achintya Dutta, Delhi, Kalpaz Publications, 2005, pp. 235-254.

125. Banerjee D. K. "Magico-religious beliefs about plants among some adibasis of India". *Journal of Mythological Sociology*, Vol. 65, No. 3, 1974, pp. 5-8.

126. Banerjee, A. K. and Banerjee, I. "A survey of the medicinal plants in Shevaroy Hills". *Journal of Economic and Taxonomic Botany*, Vol. 8, No. 2, pp. 271-290.

127. Banerjee, Archana "Medicinal uses of some flowers by Santhals of West Bengal". In Ethnobotany and medicinal plants of Indian Sub-continent, edited by J. K. Maheshwari, Jodhpur, India Scientific Publishers, 2000.

128. Banerjee, B. G. "Folk illness and ethnomedicine". New Delhi, Northern, Book Central, 1988. p.133.

129. Banerjee, D. "Place of indigenous and the western systems of medicine in the health services in India". *International Journal of Health Services*, Vol. 9, No. 3, 1979, pp. 511-519.

130. Banerjee, D. K. "Observation on the ethno-botany of Areku valley, Visakhapatnam, district, Andhra Pradesh". *Journal of Science club,* Vol. 31, No. 1, 1977, pp. 14-21.

131. Banerjee, Madhulika "Public policy and ayurveda: modernising a great tradition". *Economic and Political Weekly*, Vol. 37, No. 12, 2002, pp. 1136-1146.

132. Banerjee, P., Sahoo, K. N. and Biswas, T. K. "Bees make medicine for mankind". *Indian Journal of Traditional Knowledge,* Vol. 2, No. 1, 2003, pp. 22-26.

133. Banerjee, Parthasarathi "The traditional literacy and indigenous knowledge in colonial Bengal". *Contemporary India*, Vol. 2, No. 1, 2003, pp.157-175.

134. Banerjee, R. N. and Ghora, Chhabi "On the domestic use of some unreported plants of West Dinajpur district (West Bengal)". In Ethnobotany and medicinal plants of Indian Sub-continent, edited by J. K. Maheshwari, Jodhpur, India Scientific Publishers, 2000.

135. Banerji, Debabar "Social and cultural foundations of the health services systems of India". Centre of Social Medicine and Community Health, Jawaharlal Nehru University, New Delhi, 1974.

136. Bangwal, K. K. and Gusai, S. S. "Bhotiya janjati ke lok vishwas, bimari ka karan aour upchar". *Vanyajati*, Vol. 58, No. 1, 2010, pp. 37-43. [Hindi]

137. Bannerman, R. H. "Organization and cooperation of the development of studies on plants used in traditional medicine: some guidelines for research and studies". *Journal of Ethnopharmacology*, Vol. 2, No. 2, 1980, pp. 189-192.

138. Bannerman, Robert H., Burton, John and Wen Chieh, Ch'en (eds.) "Traditional medicine and health care coverage: A reader for health administrators and practitioners". Geneva, World Health Organization, 1983, p. 342.

139. Bannermann, R. H. "World Health Organisataion programme in traditional Medicine". *World Health Organisaton Chronicle*, Vol. 31, 1977, pp. 421-428.

140. Barbhuiya, A. R., Sharma, G. D., Arunachalam, A. and Deb, S. "Diversity and conservation of medicinal plants in Barak Valley, Northeast India". *Indian Journal of Traditional Knowledge,* Vol. 8, No. 2, 2009, pp. 169-175.

141. Bardhan, A., Dubey, D. C. and Sinha, S. K. "An exploration in utilization of modern health practices of the Bhils". In Tribal health in India, edited by Salil Basu, Delhi, Manak Publications.1994, pp. 185-195.

142. Barma, Kishore Deb "Tribal folk medicine of Tripura". Tripura, Tribal Research Institute, 1994. p. 44.

143. Barua, Saumitra "A study on indigenous health practices among the Kaman Mishmis of Lohit district of Arunachal Pradesh". *Human Science*, Vol. 33, No. 4, 1984, pp. 332-344.

144. Baruah, P. and Sharma, G. C. "Studies on the medicinal uses of plants by the Boro tribals of Assam II". *Journal of Economic and Taxonomic Botany*, Vol. 5, 1984, pp. 599-604.

145. Baruah, Parukutty and Sharma, G. C. "Studies on the

medicinal use of plants by the North East tribes-III". *Journal of Economic and Taxonomic Botany*, Vol. 11, 1987, pp. 65-70.

146. Baruah, Pixy Bhani "Traditional child care practices among the Kaibartas of North Guwahati". In Intangible Cultural Heritage of Assam, edited by Kishor. K. Basa and Brinchi K. Medhi, IGRMS, Bhopal and Pratibha Prakashan, Delhi, 2008, pp. 292-298.

147. Basa, K.K. and Medhi, Birinchi K. "Intangible cultural heritage of Assam". IGRMS, Bhopal and Pratibha Prakashan, Delhi, 2008, p. 308.

148. Basavanagoude, T. T. "Some thoughts on tribal health: A brief perspective". *Journal of Social Anthropology*, Vol. 1, No. 2, 2004, pp. 279-284.

149. Basu, B. D. (ed.) "Indian medicinal plants". Dehra Dun, Bishen Singh Mahendra Pal Singh, 1992, p. 1033.

150. Basu, Ram Sankar "Ethnobotany of the oil extraction process by the 'Santhals' of Banduan in Purulia". *Ethnobotany*, Vol. 9, No. 1-2, 1997 pp. 132-134

151. Basu, Ramsankar and Mukherjee, Prasanta Kumar "Ethnobotany of the practice of piggery by the Savars in the district of Purulia in West Bengal". In Ethnobotany and medicinal Plants of Indian Sub-continent, edited by J. K. Maheshwari, Jodhpur, India Scientific Publishers, 2000.

152. Basu, S. "Health problems of the tribal population in India". *Bulletin of the Department of Anthropology, Dibrugarh University*, Vol. 20, 1992, pp. 12-29.

153. Basu, Salil "Health and culture among the underprivileged groups in India". In State of India's health, edited by A. Mukhopadhyay, New Delhi, Voluntary Health Association of India, 1992, pp.175-188.

154. Basu, Salil (eds.) "Tribal health in India". Manak Publications, 1994, p. 349.

155. Basu, Salil, Anil Jindal, and Gautam Kshatriya "Perception of health and pattern of health seeking behaviour among the selected tribal population groups of Madhya Pradesh and Orissa". In Tribal Health in India, edited by Salil Basu, Delhi, Manak Publications 1994, pp. 26-39.

156. Basumatary, S. K. Ahmed, M. and Deka, S. P. "Some medicinal plant leaves used by Boro (tribal) people of Goalpara district, Assam". *Indian Journal of Natural Products and Resources,* Vol. 3, No. 2, 2004, pp. 88-90.

157. Baviskar, A. "Indian Indigeneities: Adivasi engagements with Hindu Nationalism in India". In Indigenous Experience today, editd by Marisol de la Cadena and Orin Starn, New York, Berg Publishers, 2007, pp. 275-303.

158. Beals, Alan R. "Strategies of resort to curers in South India". In Asian medical systems edited by Charles Leslie, 1976, Berkeley, University of California Press, pp. 184-200.

159. Bebarta, Prafulla Chandra "Concepts of disease and therapeutic practices among the Hill Saoras of Orissa". *Vanyajati*, Vol. 7, No. 2, 1959, pp. 44-48.

160. Behera, Soumit K., Panda, Anima and Behera, Susanta K. "Medicinal plants used by the Kandhas of Kandhamal district of Orissa". *Indian Journal of Traditional Knowledge,* Vol. 5, No, 4, 2006, pp. 519-528.

161. Behra, S.K. and Misra, M.K. "Indigenous phytotherapy of genito-urinary disease used by the Kandha tribe of Orissa, India". *Journal of Ethnopharmacology*, Vol. 102, 2005, pp. 319-325.

162. Bennet, S.S.R. "Ethnobotanical studies in the Nagarhaveli forests- some interesting native drugs". *Indian Forestry*, Vol. 104, 1978, pp. 676-681.

163. Bera, Sayantan "The secret garden". *Down to Earth*, Vol. 20, No.12, 2011, pp. 43-45.

164. Bhadula, S. K. and others "Distribution pattern, population diversity and propagation of some high altitude medicinal herbs from Garhwal Himalaya: Problems and prospects for conservation". In High Altitude of the Himalaya-II (Biodiversity, Ecology and Environment) edited Y. P. S. Pangety, Gyanogaya Prakasan, Nainital, pp. 389-413.

165. Bhagwat, S. and Chirmulay, D. "Traditional healing practices in rural Karnataka". *Man in India*, Vol. 77, No. 1, 1997, pp. 71-82.

166. Bhalla, N. P., Sahu, T. R., Mishra, G. P. and Dakwale, R. N. "Traditional plant medicines of Sagar District, M. P.".

Indian Journal of Economic and Taxonomic Botany, Vol. 3, No. 1, 1982, pp. 23-32.

167. Bhalla, Suman, Patel, J. R. and Bhalla P. "Ethnomedicinal observations on some asteraceae of Bundelkhand region, Madhya Pradesh". In Ethnobotany and medicinal plants of Indian Sub-continent, edited by J. K. Maheshwari, Jodhpur, India Scientific Publishers, 2000.

168. Bhandari, M. M. "Famine feeds in Rajasthan district". *Economic Botany*, Vol. 28, 1974, pp. 73-81.

169. Bhandari, M.M. "Folklore medicines and feed plants of the Indian desert". *International Congress of Anthropological and Ecological Sciences*, Vol. 2, 1978, p. 113.

170. Bhandari, Sakshi, Singh, Rana Man and Samant, S.S. "Indigenous knowledge of the medicinal plants in Kullu Valley of Northwestern Himalaya: A case - study". *Journal of Social Anthropology*, Vol. 6, No. 1-2, 2009, pp. 63-74.

171. Bhandary, M.J. and Chandrasekhar, K.R. "Treatment of poisonous snake-bite in the ethnomedicine of coastal Karnataka". *Journal of Medicinal and Aromatic Plants Science,* Vol.22, No. 4A, 2000-2001, pp. 505-510,

172. Bhandary, M. J. and Chandrashekar, K. R. "Glimpses of ethnic herbal medicine of Coastal Karnataka". *Ethnobotany*, Vol. 14, No. 1-2, 2002, pp. 1-12.

173. Bhandary, M. J. and Chandrashekar, K. R. "Herbal therapy for herbs in the ethno-medicine of coastal Karnataka". *Indian Journal of Traditional Knowledge,* Vol. 10, No, 3, 2011, pp. 528-532.

174. Bhandary, M. J., Chandrashekar, K. R. & Kaveriappa, K. M. "Ethnobotany of Gowlis of Uttara Kannada district, Karnataka". In Ethnobotany and medicinal plants of Indian Sub-continent, edited by J. K. Maheshwari, Jodhpur, India Scientific Publishers, 2000.

175. Bharadwaj, Sujata and Gakhar, S. K. "Ethnomedicinal plants used by the tribals of Mizoram to cure dysentery". *Ethnobotany*, Vol. 15, No. 1-2, 2003, pp. 51-54.

176. Bharat, K.P. and Hemant, K. B. "Ethnomedicinal plant use by Lepcha tribe of Dzongu valley, bordering Khangchendzonga Biosphere Reserve, in North Sikkim".

India Journal of Ethnobiology Ethnomedicine, Vol. 4, No. 22, 2008.

177. Bharathi, S. Bhakthavatsala "Ritual healing: Metamedical discourse and discursive practices of a south Indian nomadic sub-caste". *Man in India*, Vol. 78, No. 3-4, 1998, pp. 239-253.

178. Bharati, Kumar Avinash and Sharma, B.L. "Some ethnoveterinary plant records for Sikkim Himalaya". *Indian Journal of Traditional Knowledge,* Vol. 9, No. 2, 2009, pp. 344-346.

179. Bhardwaj, M. "Attitude Towards different systems of medicine-A survey of four villages in Punjab". In Geographical aspects of health and disease in India, edited by Akhtar Rais and A.T.A. Learmonth, New Delhi, Concept publishing company, 1985.

180. Bhargava, K. S. "Unusaul and supplementary food plants of Kumaun". *Journal of Bombay Natural History Society,* Vol. 56, 1959, pp. 26-31.

181. Bhargava, N. "Plants in folk-life and folklore in Andaman and Nicobar Islands". In Glimpses of Indian Ethnobotany, edited by S. K. Jain, 1981, pp. 329-344.

182. Bhasin, Veena "Social change, religion and medicine among Brokpas of Ladakh". *Studies on ethno-medicine*, Vol. 2, No. 2, pp. 2008, pp. 77-102.

183. Bhasin, Veena "Ecology and health: A study among tribals of Ladakh". *Studies of Tribes and Tribals*, Vol. 3, No. 1, 2005, pp. 1-13.

184. Bhasin, Veena "Gaddis' folk medicine: A source of healing". *Studies on Ethno- medicine*, Vol. 2, No. 1, 2008, pp.1-27.

185. Bhasin, Veena "Medical pluralism and health services in Ladakh". *Journal of Social Sciences*, Vol. 1, No. 1, 1997, pp. 43-69.

186. Bhasin, Veena "Traditional medicine among tribals of Rajasthan". *Journal of Social Science,* Vol. 6, No. 3, 2002, pp. 153-172.

187. Bhat, K. H. "Medicinemen of Basavanhalli: A study of Ethnomedicine". *Journal of the Indian Anthropological Society*, Vol. 2. No.1, 1976.

188. Bhat, Sathyanarayana "Folk medicine in India". In Medicine and life sciences in India edited by B. V. Subbarayappa, Delhi, Project of history of Indian science, philosophy, and culture, centre for studies in civilizations. Bharatiya Kala Prakashan, 2006, p. 294.

189. Bhatia, J. C., Dharam Vir, A. Timmappaya, and C. S. Chuttani "Traditional healers and modern medicine". *Social Science and Medicine*, Vol. 9, 1975, pp. 15-21.

190. Bhatla, N., Mukherjee, T. and Singh, G. "Plants: Trditional worshiping". *Indian Journal of History of Science*, Vol. 19, No. 1, 1984, pp. 37-42.

191. Bhatnagar, G. S. "Community responses to health: A study conducted in Patiala village in Punjab". Paper presented at the 14th All India Sociological Conference, Jabalpur University, Jabalpur, 1987.

192. Bhatt, D.C., Mehta, S.K. and Mitaliya, K.D. "Ethnomedicinal plants of Shetrunjaya hill of Palitana, Gujarat". *Ethnobotany*, Vol. 11, No. 1-2, 1999, pp. 22- 25.

193. Bhatt, D.C., Mitaliya, K.D. and Mehta, S.K. "Some sacred plants of Gujarat and ther medicinal uses". *Ethnobotany*, Vol. 13, 2001, pp. 146-149.

194. Bhatt, D.C., Mitaliya, K. D. and Mehta, S. K. "Observations on ethno veterinary herbal practices in Gujarat". *Ethnobotany*, Vol. 13, No. 1-2, 2001, pp. 91- 95.

195. Bhatt, D. C., Patel, N. K., Mitaliya, K. D. & Ant, H. M. "Herbal magic by contact therapy among tribals and rurals of Gujarat". In Ethnobotany and medicinal plants of India and Nepal edited by Singh and Jain, Scientific publishers, Jaipur, 2003, pp. 98-103.

196. Bhatt, K. C. and Gaur, R. D. "A contribution to ethnobotany of Rajis in Pithoragarh district". *Acta Botanica Indica*, Vol. 20, 1992, pp. 76-83.

197. Bhatt, K. C., Bist, M. K., Gaur, R. D. "Folk-medicines of Byans Valley in Pithoragarh". *Journal of Himalayan Studies and Regional Development*, Vol. 11, No. 12, 1987-89, p. 117-123.

198. Bhatt, K. H. "Concept of health and disease among the Pnars of Meghalaya". In Tribal health: Socio-Cultural

dimentions, edited by Buddhadeb Chaudhuri, New Delhi, Inter India, 1986, pp. 259-274

199. Bhatt, V. P. "Ethnomedicine of pilgrims at Badrinath, the holy Himalayan shrine of Hindus". In Abstract of Fourth International Congress of Ethnobiology in Human Welfare NBRI, Lucknow, India, 17-21, November 1994, p. 144.

200. Bhattacharjee, A. and Chatterjee, Soumyadip "Medicinal plants used in skin disease in Deganga, West Bengal". *Indian Journal of Traditional Knowledge,* Vol. 6, No. 2, 2007, pp. 358-359.

201. Bhattacharjee, A. K. and Pal, D. C. and Mukherjee "Diabetes and Indian tribal medicine". In Tribal health: Socio-Cultural dimentions, edited by Buddhadeb Chaudhuri, New Delhi, Inter India, 1986, pp. 333-338.

202. Bhattacharjee, S., Tiwari, K. C., Majumdar, R. & Misra, A. K. "Folklore medicine from district Kamrup (Assam)". *Bulletin of Ethno Medico Botanical Research,* Vol. 1, 1980, pp. 447-460.

203. Bhattacharjee, Supriya Kumar "Handbook of medicinal plants". Jaipur, Pointer, 1998. p. 474.

204. Bhattachary, P. and Ghatak, N. K. "Ethnobotanical aspects of spirulina: a new concept for biological treatment of anthropogenic compounds". *Folklore,* Vol. 29 No. 6, 1988, pp. 127-130.

205. Bhattacharya, A.K. (ed.) "Collected works of Benoytosh Bhattacharya: research on alternative medicine". Calcutta, Firma KLM Private, 1998, p. 330.

206. Bhattacharya, A. K. "Integrated practical and holistic medicine: a new approach". Calcutta, Firma KLM Private, 1995, p. 117.

207. Bhattacharya, S. and Sengupta, Syamal Kanti "The Concept of disease and its treatment among the Birhors of Purulia". In Tribal Health: Socio-cultural dimensions, edited by Buddhadeb Chaudhuri, New Delhi, Inter India Publications, 1986.

208. Bhattacharyyam, Goutam "Medico-ethno-botanical value of Saurashtra weeds". In Ethnobotany and medicinal plants

of Indian Sub-continent, edited by J. K. Maheshwari, Jodhpur, India Scientific Publishers, 1996, pp. 166-168.

209. Bhimaya, C. P., Bose, A. B., and Malhotra, S. P. "The Human factor in relation to trees and shrubs in a village in arid parts of Rajasthan". *Indian forestry*, Vol. 87, pp. 614-617.

210. Bhogaonkar, P. Y. and Ahmad, S. A. "Less known folklore unani uses of plants in Amravati district, Maharashtra (India)". *Ethnobotany*, Vol. 19, No. 1-2, 2007, pp. 124-127.

211. Bhogaonkar, P.Y. and Devarkar, V.D. "Some unique ethnomedicinal plants of Korkus of Melghat Tiger Reserve (Maharashtra)". *Ethnobotany*, Vol. 14, No. 1-2, 2002, pp. 16-19.

212. Bhogaonkar, P.Y. and Kadam, V.N. "Ethno-medicobotany of some local reproductive health practices in unmarked of Yavatmal district in Maharashtra, India". *Ethnobotany*, Vol. 18, No. 1-2, 2006, pp..107-113.

213. Bhowmick, P.K. "Some aspects of magico-religious beliefs and practices of Mundas". *Folklore*, Vol. 8, No. 3, 1966.

214. Bhowmick, P. K. "Treatment of disease among the Lodhas of West Bengal". *Man in India*, Vol. 35, No. 4, 1955,

215. Bhowmick, P. K. and Pal, Anadi "Indigenous health practices among Nocte of Arunachal Pradesh". *Human Science*, Vol. 33, 1984, pp. 35-53.

216. Bhowmik, Debjit and others "Traditional herbal medicines: An overview". *Archives of Applied Science Research* (Available online at www.scholarsresearchlibrary.com), Vol. 1, No. 2, 2009, pp. 165-177.

217. Billore, K. V. and Audichya, K. C. "Some oral contraceptives in family planning tribal way", *Journal of Research in Indian Medicine*, Vol. 13, No. 2, 1978, p. 104.

218. Binu Thomas, A., Rajendran, V., Aravindhan and R. Sivalingam "Ethnoveterinary medicines of tribe Paniyars in Kerala, India". *International Journal of Biological Technology*, Vol. 2, No. 2, 2011, pp. 72-75.

219. Binu, S. "Medicinal plants used for treating body pain by the tribals in Pathanamthitta district, Kerala, India". *Indian Journal of Traditional Knowledge,* Vol. 10, No. 3, 2011,

pp. 547-549.

220. Biradar, S. D. and Ghorband, D. P. "Ethnomedicinal wisdom of tribals of Kinwat forest of Nanded district (Maharashtra)". *Indian Journal of Natural Products and Resources,* Vol. 1, No. 2, 2010, pp. 254-257.

221. Bisht, Asha and Jain, S. P. "Review of Ethnobotanical Studies of Genus Rubus (Rosaceae) from North-Western Himalayas". *Ethnobotany*, Vol. 18, No. 1-2, 2006, pp. 127-130.

222. Bisht, Sudhir Singh, Buchar, S. K. & Kothyari, B. P. "Traditional skill of resource utilization". *Indian Journal of Traditional Knowledge,* Vol. 5, No. 3, 2006, pp. 403-406.

223. Bisset, Norman Grainger "Herbal drugs and phytopharmaceuticals: A handbook for practice on a scientific basis" Germany Medpharm, 2001, p. 566.

224. Bist, L. "Gheengaru: beemar dil ke leeye Himalayee tohpha". *Uttarakhand*, Vol. 8, 1994, pp. 95-98. [Hindi]

225. Bist, M. K. and Badoni, A. K. "Araceae in the folk life of tribal population in Garhwal Himalaya". *Journal of Economic Botany and Phytochemistry*, Vol. 1, 1990, pp. 21-24.

226. Bist, M. K. and others "Folk medicines of Arakot valley in District Uttarkashi: an ethnobotanical study". In Indigenous medicinal plants: including microbes and fungi edited by Purshotam Kaushik, Today and tomorrow's printers and Publishers, New Delhi, 1988, pp. 157-166.

227. Biswal, A. K. "Tribal medicine and medicine men -an exploratory study of the Bondo of Orissa and Didayi of Orissa". *Adibasi*, Vol. 37, No. 2, 1997.

228. Biswas, K. "Common medicinal plants of Darjeeling and Sikkim". Calcutta, 1956.

229. Biswas, K. and Ghosh, E. "Bharatiya Banaushodi". 2 Vols. (in Bengali), Calcutta, 1950-52.

230. Biswas, K., and Chopra, R. N. "Common medicinal plants of Darjeeling and Sikkim Himalayas". Periodical Experts Book Agency, Delhi, 1982.

231. Biswas, P. C. "Concept of disease among the primitive people of India". *Journal of Department Letters*, Vol. 25,

1934.

232. Biswas, S. "Rare and threatened taxa in the forest flora of Tehri Garhwal Himalaya and the strategy for their conservation". *Indian Journal of Forestry*, Vol. 11, 1988, pp. 233-237.

233. Blackham, Robert J. "Incomparable India: tradition, superstition, truth". Delhi, Victory Book International, 1991, p. 302.

234. Boban, Jose "Tribal ethnomedicine: Continuity and change". New Delhi, A.P.H., 1998, p. 341.

235. Bodding, Paul Olaf "Studies Santal medicine and connected folklore". Kolkata, Asiatic Society, 2001, p. 502.

236. Bodding, Paul Olaf "Studies in Santhal medicine and connected folklore II, Santals and diseases". *Memoir of Asiatic society of Bengal,* Vol, 10, No. 1, 1925, pp, 1-132.

237. Bodding, Paul Olaf "Studies in Santhal medicine and connected folklore III, The Santals and how they live". *Memoir of Asiatic society of Bengal*, Vol. 10, No. 3, 1940, pp. 427-502.

238. Bodding, Paul Olaf "The Santal Medicine" (Memoirs of Asiatic Society Bengal, Calcutta) 1927, also incorporated in the book entitled, Studies in Santal Medicine and Connected folklore (Asiatic Society Calcutta) 1986.

239. Bodeker, G. "A framework for cost-benefit analysis of traditional medicine and conventional medicine". In Traditional Medicine in Asia, edited by Ranjit Roy Chaudhury and Uton Muchtar Rafei, World Health Organization Regional Office for South-East Asia, New Delhi, 2001, pp. 159-182.

240. Bondya, S. L., Khanna, K. K. and Singh, K. P. "Ethnomedicinal uses of leafy vegetables from the tribal folk-lore of Achanakmar-Amarkantak Biosphere Reserve: (Madhya Pradesh and Chhattisgarh)". *Ethnobotany*, Vol. 18, No. 1-2, 2006, pp. 145- 148.

241. Bora, H. R. and Pandey, A. K. "Less known wild food plants of Assam". In Ethnobotany and medicinal plants of Indian Sub-continent, edited by J. K. Maheshwari, Jodhpur, India Scientific Publishers, 2000.

242. Bora, P. J. "A study on ethnomedicinal uses of plants among the Bodo tribe of Sonitpur district, Assam". In Ethnobotany and medicinal plant of Indian subcontinent, edited by J.K. Maheshwari, Saujanya Books, Jodhpur, 2003, p. 672.

243. Borah, P. K., Gogoi, P. and Phukan, A. C. "Traditional medicine in the treatment of gastrointestinal diseases in Upper Assam". *Indian Journal of Traditional Knowledge,* Vol. 5, No. 4, 2006, pp. 510-512.

244. Borah, S. and Das, A. K. "Ethnomedicinal plants used by Mishing communities for analgesic and anti-inflammatory properties in India". *Ethnobotany*, Vol. 21, No. 1-2, 2009, pp. 66- 69.

245. Borins, Mel "Traditional medicine of India". *Canadian Family Physician*, Vol. 33, April 1987, pp. 1061-1065. (http://www.ncbi.nlm.nih.gov/pmc/articles/PMC2218447/pdf/canfamphys00182-0255.pdf)

246. Borkataki, Sarat, Chutia, Mahanada and Borthakur, S. K. "Ethnobotany of biofencing among tea garden and ex-teagarden communities of Nagaon District of Assam". *Indian Journal of Traditional Knowledge,* Vol. 7, No. 4, 2008, pp. 666-668.

247. Borse, S.C., Bhamre, P. B. and Patil, D. A. "Medicinal plant lore of the tribals of Dhule (Maharashtra)". *Biojournal* Vol. 2, No. 1, 1990, pp. 47-54.

248. Borthakur, S.K. "Certain plants in folklore and folk life of Karbis (Mikirs) of Assam". In Glimpses of Indian Ethnobotany, edited by S.K. Jain, Scienific Publishers, Jodhpur, 1981, pp. 180-190.

249. Borthakur, S. K. "Less known medicinal uses of plants among the tribals of Mikir Hills". *Bulletin of the Botanical Survey of India*, Vol. 18, 1976, pp. 166-171.

250. Borthakur, S. K. "Native Phytotherapy for Child and Women Diseases from Assam". *Ethnobotany*, Vol. 5, No. 1-2, 1993, pp. 87- 91.

251. Borthakur, S.K. and Goswami, N. "Herbal remedies from Dimasa of Kamrup district of Assam in North Eastern India". *Fitoterapia*, Vol. 66, No. 4, 1995, pp. 333-339.

252. Borthakur, S. K., Choudhury, B. T. & Gogoi, R. "Folklore hepato-protective herbal recipes from Assam in Northeast

India". *Ethnobotany*, Vol. 16, No. 1-2, 2004, pp. 76-.82.

253. Brahmam, M. and Saxena, H. O. "Ethnobotany of Gandhamardan Hills: some noteworthy folk- medicinal uses". *Ethnobotany*, Vol. 2, No. 1-2, 1990, pp. 71- 79.

254. Brijlal, Upreti, D. K. and Kalakoti, B. S. "Ethnobotanical utilisation of lichens by the tribals of Madhya Pradesh (India)". *Journal of Economic and Taxonomic Botany*, Vol. 7, 1985, pp. 203-204.

255. Britto, C. A. A. "Indian Systems of Medicine and homeopathy". Bombay, Foundation for Research in Community Health, 1984.

256. Bromlei, V. and Voronov, A. A. "Folk medicine as a subject of ethnographic investigation". *Soviet Anthropology and Archaeology*, Vol. 18. No. 1, 1979, pp. 3-31.

257. Brook, Ryan K. and McLachlan, Stephane M. "Trends and prospects for local knowledge in ecological and conservation research and monitoring". *Biodiversity and Conservation*, Vol. 17, No. 14, 2008, pp. 3501-3512.

258. Brush, Stephen B. "Indigenous knowledge of biological resources and intellectual property rights: the role of anthropology". *American Anthropologist*, Vol. 95, No. 3, 1993 pp. 653-671.

259. Budd, Susan and Sharma, Ursula (ed.) "The Healing Bond: the patient-practitioner relationship and therapeutic responsibility". Routledge, London.

260. Buragohain, J. "Folk medicinal plants used in gynaecological disorders in Tinsukia district, Asssam, India". *Fitoterapia*, Vol. 79, 2008, pp. 388-392.

261. Burman, J. J. Roy "Community participation in India forestry". *Journal of Indian Anthropological Society*, Vol. 32, No. 2, 1997, pp. 173-183.

262. Burman, J. J. Roy "Ethnography of a denotified tribe: the Laman Banjara". New Delhi, Mittal Publications, 2010, p.190.

263. Burman, J. J. Roy "The dynamics of sacred groves". *Journal of Human Ecology*, Vol. 6, No. 4, 1995, pp. 245-254.

264. Burman, J. J. Roy, "Tribal medicine: traditional practices

and changes in Sikkim". New Delhi, Mittal Publications, 2003, p.165.

265. Burman, Prasenjit Deb "Disease: Is it individul or societal". In Tribal health: Socio-cultural dimentions, edited by Buddhadeb Chaudhuri, New Delhi, Inter India, 1986, pp. 185-190.

266. Burridge, W. M. "Indigenous Systems of medicine and medical research". *Indian Medical Gazette*, Vol. 62, 1927, p. 223.

267. Byg, Anja, Salick, Jan and Law, Wayne "Medicinal plant knowledge among lay people in five Eastern Tibet villages". *Human Ecology*, Vol. 38, No. 2, 2010, pp. 177-191.

268. Caius, Jean Ferdinand "Medicinal and poisonous plants of India". Jodhpur, Scientific, 1986, p. 528.

269. Carney, Louis P. "Corrections and the community". London, Prentice-Hall, 1977, p. 342.

270. Carstair, G. M. "Medicine and faith in rural Rajasthan". In Health Culture and Community, edited by B. D. Paul, New York, Russell Sage Foundations, 1955, pp. 107-135.

271. Chaghtai, S. A., Garg, A. and Ahmad, J. "Studies on the occurrence of medicinal plants of Euphorbiaceae from Bhopal and its neighbourhood". *Bulletin of Medio-Ethnobotanical Research*, Vol. 3, 1982, pp. 57-64.

272. Chaghtai, S. A., Garg, A. and Ahmad, J. "Studies on the occurrence of medicinal plants of Euphorbiaceae from Bhopal and its neighbourhood". *Nagarjun*, Vol. 22, No.4, 1978, pp. 85-87.

273. Chakrabarti, S. B. and Sarkar, B. N. "Anthropology and Medicine: An overview". *Journal of the Anthropological Survey of India*, Vol. 47, No. 3, 1998, pp. 65-77.

274. Chakraberty, Chandra "Interpretation of ancient Hindu medicine". Delhi, Low Price, 1923, p. 599.

275. Chakraborty, Aniruddha, 1986. "Some Findings on the use of Traditional Medicine in the Rural Areas of Palamau". In Tribal Health: Socio-cultural dimension, edited by Buddhadeb Chaudhuri, New Delhi, Inter-India Publications, 1986.

276. Chakraborty, M. K. and Bhattacharya, A. "Magico-religious

beliefs among the tribals of Purulia district, West Bengal". *Journal of Economic and Taxonomic Botany*, Vol. 28, 2004, pp. 510-512.

277. Champa Rani and others "Nyctanthes arbor-tristis Linn. (Night jasmine): A sacred ornamental plant with immense medicinal potentials". *Indian Journal of Traditional Knowledge,* Vol. 11, No. 3, 2012 pp. 427-435.

278. Chanda, Ranabir, Mohanty, J. P. and Bhuyun, N. R. "Medicinal plants used against gastrointestinal tract disorders by the traditional healers of Sikkim Himalayas". *Indian Journal of Traditional Knowledge,* Vol. 6, No. 4, 2007 pp. 606-610.

279. Chander, Ramesh, Khanna, A. K. and Mathur, S. K. "Antidyslipemic and antioxidant activities of SBC: A herbal preparation". *Ethnobotany*, Vol. 14, No. 1&2, 2002, pp. 123-128.

280. Chandler, R. F., Freeman, L. and Hooper, S. N. "Herbal remedies of maritime Indians". *Journal of Ethnopharmocology*, Vol. 1, 1979, pp. 49-68.

281. Chandra K, and Pandey, B. N. "Medicinal plants of Santhal Pragana district Dumka (Bihar)-Part I". *Sachitra Ayurveda,* Vol. 38, 1985, pp. 307-314.

282. Chandra K, Pandey, B. N. and Lal, V. K. "Folklore medicinal plants of Dumka (Bihar)". *Ancient Science of Life*, Vol. 4, No. 3, 1984, pp. 181-185.

283. Chandra, K. "Traditional remedies of Baharaich and Gonda District of Uttar Pradesh". *Sachitra Ayurveda*, Vol. 37, 1985, pp. 483-486.

284. Chandra, K. and Pande, H. C. "Collection of plants around Agora-Dodital in Uttar Kashi district of Uttar Pradesh, with medicinal values and folklore claims". *International Journal of Crude Drugs Research,* Vol. 21, 1983, pp. 21-28.

285. Chandra, K. and Pandey B. N. "Some folk medicines of Singhbhum (Bihar)". *Sachitra Ayurveda*, Vol. 37, 1984, pp. 253-257.

286. Chandra, Kailash "Ethno-Biological studies of the Jarawa Tribe". *Journal of the Anthropological Survey of India,* Vol. 48, No. 2, 1999, pp. 105-116.

287. Chandra, P. "Concepts of disease and theraptics practices among the Hill-Saoras of Orissa". *Vanyajati*, Vol. 7, 1957.

288. Chandra, Ramesh "Tribal health and medicine". In Tribal health and medicines, edited by A. K. Kalla and P. C. Joshi, New Delhi: Concept Publishing Co., 2004, pp. 408-415.

289. Chandra, Shailja "Role of traditional systems of medicine in national health care systems". In Traditional Medicine in Asia, edited by Ranjit Roy Chaudhury and Uton Muchtar Rafei, World Health Organization Regional Office for South-East Asia, New Delhi, 2001, pp. 135-158.

290. Chandrasekhar, K. and Srivastava, S. K. "Ethnomedicinal Studies in Pin Valley National Park, Lahaul Spiti, Himachal Pradesh". *Ethnobotany*, Vol. 15, No. 1-2, 2003, pp. 44-47.

291. Chandrasekaran, K., Ramchandran, T. and Vigneswaran, C. "Effect of medicinal herbs extracts treated garments on selected disease". *Indian Journal of Traditional Knowledge*, Vol. 11, No. 3, 2012, pp. 493-498.

292. Changikija, S. and Kumar, Y. "Ethnobotanical folk practices and beliefs of the Ao- Nagas in Nagaland, India". *Ethnobotany*, Vol. 8, 1996, pp. 26-30.

293. Charde, M. S., Hemke, A. T. and Saturwar, P. M. "Investigation on the wound healing activity of Tilvadi Ghrita: A herbal formulation". *Indian Journal of Traditional Knowledge,* Vol. 3, No. 3, 2004, pp. 247-252.

294. Chatterjee, A. and Pakrashi, S. C. (eds.) "The Treatise on Indian medicinal plants". Council of Science and Industrial Research, New Delhi, 1991.

295. Chatterjee, Kali "In search of an alternative". In State of India's Health, edited by A. Mukhopadhyay, New Delhi, Voluntary Health Association of India, 1992, pp.163-174.

296. Chattopadhyay, A. "Medicinal use of Litosa, Bhatkaiya and Behaya in Varavasi". *Nagarjun*, Vol. 25, 1982, No. 5, p. 110.

297. Chattopadhyay, A. and Maji, M. "Some medicinal trees of Bankura district of West Bengal". *Nagarjun*, Vol. 19, No. 3, 1975, p. 6.

298. Chaturvedi, G. N. "Traditional medicine: perspectives and

priorities". *Bulletin of Indian Medicine (Benares)*, 1976-77, pp. 67-68.

299. Chaturvedi, G. N. and Singh, R. H. "Treatment of Jaundice with an indigenous drug Picrorhiza Kurroa". *Current Medical Practice*, Vol. 9, 1965, pp. 451.

300. Chaturvedi, Shashank "Climate change and indigenous knowledge". *Angarag,* Issue No. 54, 2010, pp. 36-38.

301. Chaudhari, B., Dasgupta, D. and Chatterjee, K. "Tribal medicine". Regional Research and Study Centre, West Bengal, 1989.

302. Chaudhari, U. S. and Hutke, Varsha "Ethno-Medico-Botanical information on some plants used by Melghat tribes of Amravati district, Maharashtra". *Ethnobotany,* Vol. 14, No. 1-2, 2002, pp. 100-102.

303. Chaudhary, S. N. and Basa, Kishore K. (eds.) "Tribes and their indigenous knowledge: implications for development". IGRMS, Bhopal, 2008

304. Chaudhary, S. N. and Singh, R. P. "Tribals and their indigenous knowledge in agricultural management: A case study of Gond" *The Eastern Anthropologist*, Vol. 59, No. 3-4, 2006 pp. 339-417.

305. Chaudhary, S. N. and Singh, R. P. "Tribes of Pachmarhi biosphere reserve and their indigenous knowledge". IGRMS, Bhopal and Pratibha Prakashan, Delhi, 2006, p.146.

306. Chaudhuri, A. B. "Biodiversity Endangered: India's threatened wildlife and medicinal plants". Jodhpur, Scientific Publishers, 2002, p. 359.

307. Chaudhuri, B. "Magic vs. medicine in a tribal village". Adibasi, Vol. 9, 1967, pp. 3-9.

308. Chaudhuri, B. D. "Social and cultural aspects of health". *Journal of Social and Economic Studies*, Vol. 3, No. 4, 1986, pp. 379-388.

309. Chaudhuri, Buddhadeb "Cultural dimensions of health: A study on west Bengal Villages". In Tribal health: Socio-Cultural dimentions, edited by Buddhadeb Chaudhuri, New Delhi, Inter India, 1986, pp. 289-302.

310. Chaudhuri, Buddhadeb "Science in Society: The case of tribal medicine". In Tribal health and medicines, edited by A. K. Kalla and P. C. Joshi, New Delhi: Concept Publishing Co., 2004, pp. 362-375.

311. Chaudhuri, H. N. "Notes on the magico-religious beliefs about plants among the Lodhas of Midnapur, West Bengal". *Vanyajati*, Vol. 23 No. 2&3, 1975, pp. 20-22.

312. Chaudhuri, H. N. Rai and Pal, D. C. "Poor man's medicine". *Man and Life*, Vol. 2, No. 3-4, 1976, pp. 126-131.

313. Chaudhuri, H. N. Rai, Molla, H. A., Pal, D.C. and Roy, B. "Plants used in traditional medicine by some tribals of Jalpaiguri district, West Bengal". *Bulletin of the Botanical Survey of India*, Vol. 24, 1982, pp. 87-90.

314. Chaudhuri, M. K. Das and Debnath, A. "Impact of prevalent diseases among the tribes of tribal concentrated areas of West Bengal". In Tribal health: Socio- Cultural dimensions, edited by B. Chaudhuri, New Delhi, Inter India, 1986.

315. Chaudhuri, S. S. Datta "Miji-An Ethnic Group of Arunachal Pradesh: Ethno- Differentiation". *Journal of the Anthropological Survey of India*, Vol. 40, No. 1-2, 1991, pp. 103-108.

316. Chauhan, N. S. and Parmal, Y. S. "Some rare and interesting medicinal and aromatic plants of Western Himalaya". In Abstract of Fourth International Congress of Ethnobiology, 17-21 Nov., 1994 'Ethnobiology in Human Welfare' NBRI, Lucknow, India. Abstract Volume, 1994, p. 147.

317. Chauhan, N. S., Uniyal, M. R. and Sannd, B. N. "A preliminary study of the indigenous drugs used at the Tibetan Medical Centre, Dharamshala (H.P.)". *Nagarjun*, Vol. 22, No. 8, 1983, pp. 190-193.

318. Chauhan, R. S. and Nautiyal, M. C. "Seed germination and seed storage behaviour of Nardostachys jatamansi D. C. an endangered medicinal herb of high-altitude Himalaya". *Current Science*, Vol. 92, No. 11, 2007, pp. 1620-1624.

319. Chaurasia, O. P. and others "Podophyllum L.: An endangered and anticancerous medicinal plant–An overview". *Indian Journal of Traditional Knowledge,* Vol. 11, No. 2, 2012, pp. 234-241.

320. Cheape, Hugh "The red book of Appin: Medicine as magic and magic as medicine". *Folklore*, Vol. 104, No. 1-2, 1993, pp. 111-123.

321. Chelladurai, V. "Minnikizhangu- A unique folk medicinal plants from the Adivasis (tribals) of Point calimere, Tamil Nadu". *Bulletin of Medico-Ethnobotanical Research*, Vol. 4, 1983, pp. 148-153.

322. Chelladurai, V. and Subramanian, V. "Some tribal folk medicines of point Calimere (Kodikkarai) in Tamil Nadu". *Bulletin of Medico-Ethnobotanical Research*, Vol. 3, 1982, pp. 173-177.

323. Chevallier Mnimh, Andrew "The Encyclopedia of medicinal plants: A practical reference guide". London, Dorling Kindersley, 1996, p. 336.

324. Chherti, D. R., Parajuli, P. and Subba, G. C. "Antidiabetic plants used by Sikkim and Darjeeling Himalayan tribes, India". *Journal of Ethnopharmacology*, Vol. 99, 2005, pp. 199-202.

325. Chhetri, D. R. "Ethnomedicinal plants of the Khangchendzonga National Park, Sikkim, India". *Ethnobotany*, Vol. 17, No. 1-2, 2005, pp. 96-103.

326. Chhetri, D. R. "Medicinal plants used as antipyretic agents by the traditional healers of Darjeeling Himalayas". *Indian Journal of Traditional Knowledge,* Vol. 3, No. 3, 2004, pp. 271-275.

327. Chhetri, D. R., Basnet, Deewa and Chiu, Po fong "Current status of ethnomedicinal plants in the Darjeeling Himalaya". *Current Science*, Vol. 89, No. 2, 2005, pp. 264-368.

328. Chhetri, R. B. "Further observations on ethnomedicobotany of Khasi Hills in Meghalaya, India". *Ethnobotany*, Vol. 6, No. 1-2, 1994, pp. 33-36.

329. Chhetri, R. B. "Trends in ethnodomestication of some wild plants in Meghalaya, Northeast India". *Indian Journal of Traditional Knowledge,* Vol. 5, No. 3, 2006, pp. 342-347.

330. Chiej, Roberto "Macdonald encyclopedia of medicinal plants". London, Macdonald Book, 1984, p. 447.

331. Choondal, Chummar "Some folk medicines for Liverstock

in Kerala: an interdisciplinary approach of study is necessary". *Folklore*, Vol. 29, No. 9, 1988, pp. 193-201.

332. Chopra, I. C., Handa, K. L. & Kapur, L. D. "Indigenous Drugs of India". U. N. Dhur & Sons, Calcutta, 1958.

333. Chopra, R. N. "Supplement to glossary of Indian medicinal plants". New Delhi, Publication and Information Directorate, 1969, p. 119.

334. Chopra, R. N. "Glossary of Indian medicinal plants". New Delhi, Council of Scientific and Industrial Research, 1956, p. 330.

335. Chopra, R. N. and Chopra, I. C. "A review of work on Indian medicinal plants". New Delhi, ICAR, 1955.

336. Chopra, R. N. and Ghosh, S. "Observation on certain medicinal plants used in indigenous medicine", *Indian Journal of Medical research*, Vol. 17, 1929-30, p. 377.

337. Choudhury A. K. and Khashmisi, M. H. R. "Indigenous health practices and its problems: a study among Bhoskas of Nainital". In Education and health problems in tribal development: a study of National integration edited by Kanchan Roy, Concept Publishing House, 1989, pp. 97-102

338. Choudhury, Buddhadeb (ed.) "Cultural and environmental dimensions on health". New Delhi, Inter-India, 1990, p. 470.

339. Choudhury, Buddhadeb (ed.) "Tribal health: Socio-culture dimensions". New Delhi, Inter -India Publications, 1986, p. 350.

340. Choudhury, M. Dutta, Shil, Sanjib and Chakraborty, Gouri "Ethno-medicobotanical studies on dimasa kachari of Cachar district, Assam". *Ethnobotany*, Vol. 20, No. 1&2, 2008, pp. 128-132.

341. Choudhury, P. C. Roy "Folk-lore in aid of medicine". *Folklore*, Vol. 4, No. 9, 1963, pp. 308-309

342. Choudhury, S. S. Datta "Herbal medicine and its implications in family planning: a study based upon Singpho of Arunachal Pradesh". *Human Science*, Vol. 34, 1985, pp. 75-77.

343. Chouhan, N. S. "Medicinal and Aromatic plants of Himachal Pradesh". Indus Publishing Company, New Delhi, 1999.

344. Chouhan, Narayan Singh "Ethnobotanical study of medicinal plants of Himachal Pradesh". In Indigenous medicinal plants: including microbes and fungi edited by Purshotam Kaushik, Today and tomorrow's printers and Publishers, New Delhi, 1988, pp. 187-198.

345. Chowdhuri, Nupur "Patents bill: Protecting indigenous knowledge". *Economic and Political Weekly*, Vol. 39, No. 46-47, 2004, pp. 4984-4986.

346. Chunekar, K. C. "Rasaayana therapy of ayurveda-an eye-witness account of Kayakalpa". *Indian Journal of Traditional Knowledge,* Vol. 1, No. 1, 2002, pp. 11-16.

347. Colonel, Herber Drury "Useful plants of India". Periodical Experts Book Agency, New Delhi, 1978.

348. Coon, Carleton, S. "The hunting peoples". Toronto, Little, Brown & Company, 1971, p. 413.

349. Coreil, Jeannine "Innovation among Haitian healers: The adoption of oral rehydration therapy". *Human Organization*, Vol. 47, No. 1, 1988, pp. 48-57.

350. Correa, Carlos M. "Protection of traditional systems of medicine, patenting and promotion of medicinal plants". In Traditional Medicine in Asia, edited by Ranjit Roy Chaudhury and Uton Muchtar Rafei, World Health Organization Regional Office for South-East Asia, New Delhi, 2001, pp. 227-246.

351. Coulehan, J. L., "Indian Medicine: Implication for healing". *The Journal of Family Practice*, Vol. 10, No. 1, 1980, pp. 55-61.

352. Crevello, Stacy "Dayak land use systems and indigenous knowledge". *Journal of Human Ecology*, Vol. 16, No. 1, 2004, pp. 69-73.

353. Croley, T. K. "In the land of hostle Jarawa and other wild tribes of the Andamans". *Indian Forester*, Vol. 84, 1958, p. 449.

354. Cumston, Charles Greene "History of medicine: from the time of the pharaohs to the end of the 18th century". New Delhi, Gyan, 1999, p. 390.

355. Dabas, Kiran, Parabia, Minoo and Dabas, Jayaprakash "Cultivation and food habits of tribals of Dangs district in

Gujarat: a case study". *Ethnobotany* Vol. 2, No. 1-2, 1990, pp. 61-65.

356. Dabral, S. P. "Uttarakhand Ke pashu upchaarak". Doggada, Garhwal, 1964. [Hindi]

357. Dagar, H. S. "Euphorbiaceae in folk life of the Nicobarese tribal". *Bulletin of Medico-ethno-botanical Research*, Vol. 9, 1988, pp. 21-27.

358. Dagar, H. S. "Plant folk medicines among Nicobarese tribals of Car Nicobar Island, India". *Economic Botany*, Vol. 43, 1989, pp. 215-224.

359. Dagar, H. S. "Plants in folk medicines of the Nicobarese of Bompoka Island". *Journal of Andaman Science Association*, Vol. 5, No. 1, 1989, pp. 169-170.

360. Dagar, H. S. and Dagar, J. C. "Ethnobotanical studies of the Nicobarese of Chowra island of Nicobar group of Islands". In Ethnobotany and Medicinal Plants of Indian Sub-continent, edited by J. K. Maheshwari, Jodhpur, India Scientific Publishers, 2000.

361. Dagar, H. S. and Dagar, J. C. "Plant folk medicines among the Nicobarese of Katchal Island". *Economic Botany*, Vol. 45, No.1, 1991, pp. 114-119.

362. Dagar, H. S. and Dagar, J. C. "Plant folk medicines for gynaecological urino-genital and other related problems among aborigines of Andaman and Nicobar Islands", In Ethnobotany and medicinal plant of Indian subcontinent, edited by J. K. Maheshwari, Saujanya Books, Jodhpur, 2003, p. 672.

363. Dam, D. P. and Hazra, P. K. "Observation on ethnobotany of the Monpas pf Kemeng district Arunachal Pradesh" In Glimpses of India Ethnobotany, edited by S. K. Jain, New Delhi, Oxford & IBH 1981, pp. 107-114.

364. Dangwal, L. R. and Sharma, Antima "Indigenous traditional knowledge recorded on some medicinal plants in Narendra Nagar Block (Tehri Garhwal), Uttarakhand". *Indian Journal of Natural Products and Resources*, Vol. 2, No. 1, 2011, pp. 110-115.

365. Dangwal, L. R., Rana, C. S. and Sharma, Antima "Ethno-medicinal plants from transitional zone of Nanda Devi

Biosphere Reserve, District Chamoli, Uttarakhand (India)". *Indian Journal of Natural Products and Resources*, Vol. 2, No. 1, 2011, pp. 116-120.

366. Das Gupta, Pranab Kumar "Life and culture of matrilineal tribe of Meghalaya". New Delhi, Inter- India Publications, 1984, p. 210.

367. Das, A. K. "Less-Known Uses of Plants among the Adis of Arunachal Pradesh". *Ethnobotany*, Vol. 9, No. 1-2, 1997, pp. 90-93.

368. Das, A. K. and Saikia, D. C. "Indigenous practice of treating Human Liver Disorders in Assam". *Ethnobotany*, Vol. 13, No. 1-2, 2001, pp. 87-90.

369. Das, A. K. and Saikia, D. C. "Investigation into the Folk Belief on Anti-Fertility and fertility-Induced Plants". *Ethnobotany*, Vol. 14, No. 1-2, 2002, pp. 20-22.

370. Das, A. K. and Tag, Hui "Ethnomedicinal studies of the Khamti tribe of Arunachal Pradesh". *Indian Journal of Traditional Knowledge,* Vol. 5, No. 5, 2006, pp. 317-322.

371. Das, Achintya Kumar, Shome, Jayasri and Ghosh, Ashok K."Disease and medicinal plants in some tribal areas". *Human Science*, Vol. 35, No. 4, 1986, pp. 279-285.

372. Das, Ajit Kumar, Dutta, B. K. and Sharma, G. D. "Medicinal usede by different tribes of Cachar district, Assam". *Indian Journal of Traditional Knowledge,* Vol. 7, No. 3, 2008, pp. 446-456.

373. Das, Dhrubananda "Asomor swasthya parampara: a book on various medicines, mantras etc. of Assamese people collected and written". Guwahati, Dhrupad, 2001, p. 255.

374. Das, Farida Ahmed, Barua, Indira and Das, Deepanjana Dutta "Ethno-medicinal practices: A case study among the Sonowal Kacharis of Dibrugarh, Assam". *Studies on Ethno-medicine*, Vol. 2, No. 1, 2008, pp. 33-37.

375. Das, H. S., Panda, P. C. & Patnaik, S. N. "Traditional uses of wetland plants of Eastern Orissa". In Ethnobotany and medicinal plants of Indian sub-continent, edited by J. K. Maheshwari, Jodhpur, India Scientific Publishers, 2000.

376. Das, K. "The plant in Orissian folklore". *Folklore*, Vol. 5, 1964, pp. 187-196.

377. Das, M. "Disease and illness and their ethnomedical treatment among the Rathwas of Suskal Gujarat". In Tribal health and medicines, edited by A.K. Kalla and P.C. Joshi, New Delhi, Concept Publishing Co., 2004, pp. 283-300.

378. Das, M. B. and Sharma, T. C. "Traditional methods of treatment of leprosy among Mikirs". *Adibasi*, Vol. 3, No. 1, 1958-59, pp. 25-30.

379. Das, Mitoo "Diseases and illness and their ethnomedical treatment among the Rathwas of Suskal Gujarat". In Tribal health and medicines, edited by A. K. Kalla and P.C. Joshi, New Delhi: Concept Publishing Co., 2004, pp. 283-300.

380. Das, P. K. and Misra, M. K. "Some medicinal plants among Kondhas around Chandrapur (Koraput)". *Journal of Economic and Taxonomic Botany*, Vol. 12, 1988, pp. 103-109.

381. Das, P. K. and Misra, M. K. "Some medicinal plants used by the tribals of Deomali and adjascent areas of Koraput district, Orissa". *Indian Journal of Forestry*, Vol. 10, 1987, pp. 301-303.

382. Das, Paushali "Wild edible plants of Tripura tribes". Agartala, Tripura Tribal Cultural Research Institute and Museum, 1997, p. 146.

383. Das, S. K. "Medicinal, economic and useful plants of India". Calcutta, 1923.

384. Das, S., Dash, S.K. and Padhy S.N. "Ethnomedicine information from Orissa state, India-A review". *Journal of Human Ecology*, Vol. 14, 2003, pp. 165-227.

385. Das, Samares Kumar and Tripathi, Hema "Ethnoveternary practices and socio-cultural values asociated with animal husbandry in rural Dunderbans, West Bengal". *Indian Journal of Traditional Knowledge,* Vol. 8, No. 2, 2009, pp. 201-205.

386. Dash, Jagannath, "The concept and treatment of disease in tribal Orissa". In Tribal health: Socio-cultural dimentions, edited by Buddhadeb Chaudhuri, New Delhi, Inter India Publications, 1986,

387. Dash, P. K., Dhal, N. K. and Rout, N. C. "Pyto-therapeutic uses of mangroves for primary healthcare the local

inhabitants of Bhitarkanika Wildlife Sanctuary, Orissa, India". *Ethnobotany*, Vol. 19, No. 1-2, 2007, pp. 49-54.

388. Dash, S. S. and Misra, M. K. "Tribal uses of plants from Narayanapatnam region of Koraput district, Orissa". Ancient Science of Life, Vol. 15, 1996, pp. 230.-237.

389. Dash, Santosh Kumar and Padhy, Sachidananda "Review on ethnomedicines for diarrhea diseases from Orissa: Prevalence versus culture". *Journal of Human Ecology*, Vol. 20, No. 1, 2006, pp. 59-64.

390. Dash, Vaidya Bhagwan "Diagnosis and treatment of diseases in ayurveda: based on ayurveda saukhyam of Todarananda". New Delhi, Concept, 1991, p. 608.

391. Dash, Vaidya Bhagwan "Five specialised therapies of ayurveda (Pancha-Karma): based on ayurveda saukhyam of Todarananda". New Delhi, Concept, 1992, p. 399.

392. Dash, Vaidya Bhagwan "Materia medica of Indo-Tibetan medicine". Delhi, Classics India, 1989. p. 647.

393. Dastur, J. F. "Medicinal plants of India and Pakistan". Bombay, 1962.

394. Datt, B. and Lal, B. "Less known medicinal uses of some plants from Pithoragharh district of Kumaun Himalaya, U.P.". *Aryavaidyan,* Vol. 6, 1993, pp. 242-246.

395. Datta, S. K. "Marketing of wild medicinal plants: Tribal economy in India". *Economic and Political Weekly*, Vol. 36, No. 38, 2001, 3598-3602.

396. Datta, S. K. and others "Ethnobotany of some important medicinal plants used by the tribals of Birbhum and Bankura districts with special references to histo-chemistry and UV florescence nature of rude drugs". *SEBS, New Letter (Abstract),* Vol. 2, No.1, 1982, p. 4.

397. Datta Choudhary, S. S. "Indigenous health practices among the Idu Mishmis of Arunachal Pradesh". *Human Science,* Vol. 33, No. 1, 1984, pp. 24-34.

398. David, J. P. "Medicines and men of influence". *Man,* Vol. 3, 1968, pp. 424-439.

399. De Lazlo, H. and P. S. Hanshaw "Plants materials used by primitive peoples to affect fertility". *Science,* Vol. 119, 1954, pp. 626-623.

400. De, A. C. "Folk-lore of medicinal plants of Bhagirathi Valley (Himalaya)". Colombo, Govt. Press, Ceylon, 1962.

401. Deb, Sourabh, Arunachalam, A. and Das, A. K. "Indigenous knowledge of Nyishi tribes on traditional agroforestry systems". *Indian Journal of Traditional Knowledge,* Vol. 8, No. 1, 2009, pp. 41-46.

402. Debnath, Debashis "Indigenous knowledge in natural resource management towards tribal development". *Man and Life*, Vol. 28, No. 1-2, 2002, pp. 122-138.

403. Deka, Dipali and Sarma, Gajen Chandra "Traditionally used herbs in the preparation of rice-beer by the Rabha tribe of Goalpara district, Assam". *Indian Journal of Traditional Knowledge,* Vol. 9, No. 3, 2010, pp. 459-462.

404. Deka, M. K., Bhuyan, M. and Hazarika, L. K. "Traditional pest management practices of Assam". *Indian Journal of Traditional Knowledge,* Vol. 5, No. 1, 2006, pp. 75-78.

405. Dennehy, H. G. "Naga Medicine". *Man in India*, Vol. 7, No. 2&3, 1927, pp. 63-68.

406. Densmore, F. "How Indians use wild plants for food, medicine & crafts". New York, Dover Publications, 1974.

407. Deogaonkar, Shashishekhar Gopal and Deogaonkar, Shailaja Shashishekhar "The Banjara (volume 3 of Castes and tribes of India)". Concept Publishing Company, 1992, p. 115.

408. Desai, Prakash N. "Health and medicine in the Hindu tradition: Continuity and cohesion". New York, Crossroad Publishing, 1980.

409. Deshmukh, V. R, Muratkar, G. D., Rothe, S. P."Preliminary observation on the medicinal and economically important leguminous plant species from Amravati Tahsil", In Ethnobotany and medicinal plant of Indian subcontinent, edited by J. K. Maheshwari, Saujanya Books, Jodhpur, 2003, p. 672.

410. Deshpande, D. J. "Medicinal plants and their uses". *Udhamita Yearly,* 1998, pp. 105-108.

411. Devangan, I. L. "Pramparagat ausadhi". *Chaumasa*, Vol. 14, No. 45, 1998, pp. 117- 120. [Hindi]

412. Devaraj, T. L. "Speaking of ayurvedic remedies for common diseases". New Delhi, Sterling, 1985, p. 152.

413. Devarapali, Jesurathnam and Kumar, R. Yathiraj "Ethnomedicine: The application of plant and animal products among Chenchus". *Indian Anthropologist*, Vol. 28, No. 2, 1998, pp. 73-80.

414. Devi, J. and Borgohain, R. "Indigenous leafy vegetables of Assam: sources of nutrition and ethnomedicine". *Asian Agri-History* Vol. 16, No. 1, 2012, pp. 83-91.

415. Devi, L. D. "Ethnobiological studies of Manipur valley with reference to Museological aspects". Unpublished Ph.D. Thesis, Manipur University, 1989.

416. Devi, L. Dhanapati "Ethnobiological information of medicinal fishes in Manipur"., 4th Annual Conferene, National Environmental Science Academy, New Delhi, 1988.

417. Devi, L. Dhanapati "Ethnobotanical study of bamboo in Manipur". *Journal of Museum Association of India*, New Delhi, 1989.

418. Devi, L. Dhanapati "Folklore medicinal animals, their role in ethnobiological museum". 76th Session of Indian Science Congress Association, Anthropological and Archaeological section, Madurai, 1989.

419. Devi, L. Dhanapati "Folklore medicines of ethnobiological importance in Manipuri, (Vol. 1)". Imphal, L. D. Devi, 1990, p. 142.

420. Devi, L. Dhanapati "Medicinal plants of Manipur". *Manipur Univeristy Museum Bulletin*, Vol. 3, 1988, pp. 19-25.

421. Devi, L. Dhanapati "Medicinal plants their role in Ethnobiological museum Botany section". 76th Session of Indian Science Congress, Madurai, 1989.

422. DeWalt, Billie R. "Using indigenous knowledge to improve agriculture and natural resource management". *Human Organization*, Vol. 53 No. 2, 1994, pp. 123-131.

423. Dey, A. C. "Indian medicinal plants used in Ayurvedic prepration". Bishen Singh Mahendra Pal Singh, Dehradun, 1980.

424. Dey, Kanny Loll "The indigenous drugs of India; or Short

descriptive notices of the medicines, both vegetable and mineral in common use among the natives of India". Calcutta, Thacker, Spink & Co., 1867.

425. Dhakal, M. R. "Ayurveda: How long it will survive?". *Current Science*, Vol. 90, No. 8, 2006, p. 1052.

426. Dhal, N. K, Rout, N. C. and Thirunavoukkarasu, M. "Plumbago Indica Linn. (Plumbaginaceae): a specific case study for birth control among the Jani tribe of Orissa". *Ethnobotany*, Vol. 12, No. 1-2, 2000, pp. 27-28.

427. Dhar, U. and others "Current status and future strategy for development of medicinal plants sector in Uttaranchal, India". *Current Science*, Vol. 83, No. 8, 2002, pp. 956-964.

428. Dhar, U., Rawal, R. S. and Samant, S. S. "Wild plant resources and inhabitants in Askot Wildlife Sanctuary of Kumaun in Indian Himalaya: Conservation issue". In Biodiversity Conservation in Managed and Protected Areas, edited by P. C. Kotwal and S. Banerjee, Asro Botanica, Bikaner, 1998, pp. 128-142.

429. Dhar, V., Samant, S. S., Rawal, R. S. & Sharma, S. "Studies on biota and resource use pattern of the natives within Askot Wild Life Sanctuary of Kumaun Himalaya". *Tiger Paper*, Vol. 24, No. 4, 1997, pp. 12-18.

430. Dhasmana, H. "Medicinal plants of Pauri town (Garhwal) and adjacent forest region (Part 1: family-Compositae)". *Journal of Science Research Plant Medicine*, Vol. 7, 1986, pp. 45-49.

431. Dhasmana, H. "Medicinal plants of Pauri town and adjacent forest region (Pauri Garhwal)". *Journal of Science Research Plant Medicine*, Vol. 8, 1987, pp. 1-8.

432. Dheeman, Dila Ram "Himalaya Ki vanaushadhi Sampada". Somsi, Vol. 3 No. 1 1977, pp. 77-78.

433. Dhiman A. K. "Notes on ethnomedicinal uses of important fabaceous plants in India". *Aryavaidyan*, Vol. 13, 1999, pp. 22-29.

434. Dhiman A. K. and Kaushik, P. "Medicinal uses of some spice plants as in ancient literature". In Recent trends in spices and medicinal plants research edited by A.K. De, Associated Publishing Com., New Delhi, 2000, pp. 19-26.

435. Dhiman, Anil K. "Sacred Plants and Their Medicinal Uses". Delhi, Daya Publishing House, 2003. p. 237.

436. Dixit, A. K., Kadavul, K. and Rajalakshmi, S. "Ethno-medico-biological studies of South India". *Indian Journal of Traditional Knowledge,* Vol. 9, No. 1, 2010, pp. 116-118.

437. Dixit, R. D. and Mishra, R. "Studies on ethnobotany-II on some less known medicinal plants of Ajmer forest division, Rajasthan". *Nagarjun*, Vol. 19, 1976, pp. 20-22.

438. Dixit, R. D., Das, A. and Kar, B. D. "Studies on ethnobotany -III on some less known edible economic and medicinal ferns of Darjeeling district, West Bengal". *Nagarjun*, Vol. 21, No. 10, 1978, pp. 1-4.

439. Dixit, Rajani "Mastisk ki bimariyo ke liye harbal ausadhiyo par shodh". *Ojaswani*, April, 2010, p. 59. [Hindi]

440. Djurfeldt, G. and Lindberg, S. "Pills against poverty a study of the introduction on western medicine in a Tamil village". Lund Curjon Press, 1975.

441. Dolui, A. K., Sharma, H. K. and Marein, Theresia Breen "Folk herbal remedies from Meghalaya". *Indian Journal of Traditional Knowledge,* Vol. 3, No. 4, 2004, pp. 358-364.

442. D'Souza, Marie "Tribal medicine". Society for Promotion of Wastelands Development, New Delhi, 1993, p. 371.

443. Dube, Nidhi "Naveen ausadhiya yani new drugs". *Vigyan Pragati,* Vol. April, 2012, pp. 5-13. [Hindi]

444. Dubey, G. Shahu, P. and Sahu, R. "Role of plants in different religious ceremonies common to Bundelkhand regions of Madhya Pradesh". *Journal of Medicinal Arometic plants Science,* Vol. 22/23, No. 4A/1A, 2000-2001, pp. 542-545.

445. Dubos, R. "Man, medicine and environment". New York, Mentor.

446. Duffin, Jacalyn "History of medicine: a scandalously short introduction". Canada, University of Toronto Press, 1999, p. 432.

447. Duhoon, S. S., Koppar, M. N. & Umesh Chandra "Seabuck thorn (Hippophae spp.)-a less known wonder plant of ethno-medico-botanical importance in cold desert of India". In Ethnobotany and Medicinal Plants of Indian Sub-continent,

edited by J. K. Maheshwari, Jodhpur, India Scientific Publishers, 2000.

448. Duke, James A. "The Green Pharmacy". Jodhpur, Scientific publishers, 2002. p. 508.

449. Dunn, F. L. "Traditional Asian medicine and cosmopolitan medicine as adoptive system". In Asian medical systems: a comparative study, edited by C. Leslie, 1976, pp. 133- 158.

450. Dutt, U. C. "Materia medica of the Hindus". Delhi, Mittal Publications, 1989, p. 356.

451. Dutta, B. K. and Dutta, P. K. "Potential of ethnobotanical studies in North East India: An overview". *Indian Journal of Traditional Knowledge,* Vol. 4, No. 1, 2005, pp. 7-14.

452. Dutta, Bimal Chandra "Some observations on the diseasez and traditional medicines of the Singphos". *Man in India,* Vol. 79, No. 1-2, 1999, pp. 179-189.

453. Dutta, Gouri Pada "Non-codified medicine". *Journal of Indian Anthropological Society*, Vol. 45, No. 2, 2010, pp. 115-121.

454. Dutta, Malakshmi and Nath, Subhan C. "Ethno-medico botany of the Tai-Ahoms of Assam, India". In Ethnobotany and medicinal plant of Indian subcontinent, edited by J. K. Maheshwari, Saujanya Books, Jodhpur, 2003, p. 672.

455. Dutta, Rajeep and Bhattachariya, Birendra Kumar "An indigenous commnity fishing practice of Tiap district, Arunachal Pradesh". *Indian Journal of Traditional Knowledge,* Vol. 7, No. 4, 2008, pp. 624-626.

456. Dwarakan, P. and Alagesaboopathi, C "Traditional crude drug resources used for human and live-stock diseases in Salem district, Tamil Nadu". In Ethnobotany and medicinal plant of Indian subcontinent, edited by J. K. Maheshwari, Saujanya Books, Jodhpur, 2003, p. 672.

457. Dwarakan, P. and Ansari, A. A. "Less known uses of plants of Kollimalai (Salem distt. Tamil Nadu) in South India". In Ethnobotany and Medicinal Plants of Indian Sub-continent, edited by J. K. Maheshwari, Jodhpur, India Scientific Publishers, 2000.

458. Dwivedi, S. N. Dwivedi, Sangeeta Patel, P. C. "Medicinal plants used by the tribal and rural people of Satna district,

Madhya Pradesh for the treatment of gastrointestinal diseases and disorders". *Natural Product Radiance*, Vol. 5, No. 1, 2006, pp. 60-63.

459. Dwivedi, S. N., Dwivedi, Sangeeta & Patel, P. C. "Antimicrobial herbs used among the tribal and rural communities". *Ethnobotany*, Vol. 19, No. 1-2, 2007, pp. 111-115.

460. Eisler, Laurie "Kalaripayyat: Traditional techniques". *Discover India*, Vol. 5, No. 6, 1992, pp. 56-59.

461. Ekka Amia "Some traditional medicine for anti-fertility used by the tribals in Chhattisgarh India". *International Journal of Biology, Pharmacy and allied Science*, Vol. 1, No. 2, 2012. pp. 108-112.

462. Elanchezhian, R. and others "Ethnobotany of Shompens- a primitive tribe of Great Nicobar Island". *Indian Journal of Traditional Knowledge,* Vol. 6, No. 2, 2007, pp. 342-345.

463. Emanuel, A. E. L. "The Tulsi plant: Anthropological scraps". *Journal of Anthropological Sociology Bombay*, Vol. 8, 1907, pp. 72-80.

464. Ernst, Waltraud, (ed.) "Beyond East and West: From the History of Colonial Medicine to the Social History of Medicine(s) in South Asia". *Social History of Medicine*, Vol. 20, No. 3, 2007, pp. 505-524.

465. Ethoven R. E. "Tree and animal worship in Western India". Proceedings of Jubilee Congress- 1926, London, 1930, pp. 181-187.

466. Etkin, Nina L. "Ethnopharmacology: behavioural approaches in the anthropological Study of indigenous medicines". *Annual Review of Anthropology,* Vol. 17, 1988, pp. 23-42.

467. Fabricant, D. S. and Farnsworth, N. R. "The value of plants used in traditional medicine for drug discovery" *Environmental Health perspectives (supplement)* Vol. 109, 2001, pp. 69-75.

468. Fargusaon, J. "Tree and serpent worship". Delhi, Oriental Publishers, 1971.

469. Farooquee, Nehal A. "Indigenous ethnoveterinary knowledge and livestock management amongst

transhumant pastoralists of central Himalaya". *The Journal of Human Ecology*, Vol. 11, No. 5, 2000, pp. 319-322.

470. Farooquee, Nehal A., Majila, B. S. and Kala, C. P. "Indigenous knowledge systems and sustainable management of natural resources in a high altitude society in Kumaun". *The Journal of Human Ecology*, Vol. 16, No. 1, 2004 pp. 33-42.

471. Farooqui, M. I. H. "Plants of the Quran". Sidrah Publishers, Lucknow, 1989.

472. Fatima, Waseem "Roghara parve: A festival or a custom related to health and pollution among Mundas". *Studies on Ethno-medicine*, Vol. 6, No. 1, 2012, pp. 35-38.

473. Fernie, W. T. "Herbal simples: Approved for modern uses of cure (in 2 Vols.)". New Delhi, Logos Press, p. 651.

474. Filliozat, J. "Classical doctrine of Indian medicine: its origins and its Greek Parallels". Delhi, Munshiram Manoharlal, 1964, p. 298.

475. Fonning, A. R. "Lepcha–my vanishing tribe". Sterling Publishers Pvt. Ltd., New Delhi, India, 1987.

476. Foster, G. M. "An introduction to ethnomedicine". In Traditional Medicine and Health care coverage edited by R. H. Bannermann et al, Geṇeva, World Health Organisation, 1983.

477. Foster, G. M. "Anthropological research perspectives for medical anthropologists". *Social Science Medicine*, Vol. 18, 1984, pp. 847-854.

478. Foster, G. M. and Anderson, B. G. "Medical anthropology". New York, John Wiley & Sons, 1978.

479. Frawley, David "Ayurvedic healing: a comprhensive guide". Delhi, Motilal Banarsidass, 1989, p. 368.

480. Freeman, E. Levine Sand and Reeder, L. G. "Handbook of medical sociology". New Jersey, Englewood Cliffs, Prentice Hall, 1972.

481. Freeman, Howard E. (ed.) "Hand book of medical sociology". New Jersey, Prentice Hall, 1963, p. 548.

482. Fuchs, S. "The Gond and Bhumia of eastern Mandla". New York, Asia Publishing House, 1960.

483. Fuchus, Stephen "The Balatrus in central India". In Magic Faith and healing edited by Arikiev, Glenoe, Free Press, 1964.

484. Gadgil, Madhav "Biodiversity: Tapping folk knowledge". *The Hindu*, Jan. 10, 1993.

485. Gadgil, Madhav and Vartak, V. D. "Sacred groves in India: A plea for continuous conservation". *Journal of Bombay Natural History Society*, Vol. 72, 1976, pp. 314-320.

486. Gajurel, P. R., Rethy, P. and Singh, B. "Ethnobotanical studies on Adi tribes in Dehang Debang Biosphere Reserve in Arunachal Pradesh, Eastern Himalaya". *Ethnobotany*, Vol.18, No. 1-2, 2006, pp. 114-118.

487. Galav, P. K., Nag, Ambika and Katewa, S. S. "Traditional herbal veterinary medicines from Mount Abu, Rajasthan". *Ethnobotany*, Vol. 19, No. 1-2, 2007, pp. 120-123.

488. Ganasan, S., Chandhirasekaran, M. and Selvaraj, A. "Ethnoveterinary healthcare practices in Southern districts of Tamil Nadu". *Indian Journal of Traditional Knowledge,* Vol. 7, No. 2, 2008, pp. 347-354.

489. Gandhi, M. K. "Nature care" edited by Kumarappa, Ahmedabad, 1954.

490. Ganesan, S., Suresh, N. and Kesaven, L. "Ethnomedicinal survey of lower Palni hills of Tamil Nadu". *Indian Journal of Traditional Knowledge,* Vol. 3, No. 3, 2004, pp. 299-304.

491. Ganesan, S., Venkateshan, G. and Banumathy, N. "Medicinal plants used by ethnic group thottianaickans of semmalai hills (reserved forest), tiruchirappalli district". *Indian Journal of Traditional Knowledge,* Vol. 5, No. 2, 2006, pp. 245-252.

492. Gangadharan, G. G. "Potential of Traditional Knowledge in the development of healthcare products". *Indian Journal of Traditional Knowledge,* Vol. 4, No. 2, 2005, pp. 132-138.

493. Gangadharan, G. G. and Shankar, Darshan "Medical pluralism - The challenges ahead". *Indian Journal of Traditional Knowledge,* Vol. 8, No. 2, 2009, pp. 181-184.

494. Garbyal, S. S., Aggarwal, K. K.and Babu, C. R.

"Traditionally used medicinal plants in Dharchula Himalayas of Pithoragarh district, Uttaranchal". *Indian Journal of Traditional Knowledge,* Vol. 4, No. 2, 2005, pp. 199-207.

495. Garbyal, S. S., Grover, A. and Aggarwal, K. K. "Traditional phytomedicinal knowledge of Bhotias of Dharchula in Pithoragarh". *Indian Journal of Traditional Knowledge,* Vol. 6 No. 2, 2007, pp. 360-364.

496. Gare, G. M. and Sirsalkar, P. R. "Traditional Medicines-Ethno Botonical analysis". *Tribal Research Bulletin, Maharashtra,* Vol. 5, No. 1, 1982, pp. 13-14.

497. Garg, B. S. and Singh, J. V. "Belief about causation of diseases and preference of utilization of health agencies by elderly persons in an urban community". *Health and Population Perspectives and issues,* Vol. 8, No. 1, 1985, pp. 5-11.

498. Gaur, D. S. and Gupta, L. P. "A study on drug evaluation in ancient India". In Advances in Research in India Medicines Varanasi, 1970.

499. Gaur, Mokshika "Forest and the notion of health among Korwa of Chhattisgarh". *Journal of Indian Anthropological Society,* Vol. 40, No. 1, 2005, pp. 51-64.

500. Gaur, R. D. "A contribution to the flora of Srinagar Garhwal". *Journal of Economic and Taxonomic Botany,* Vol. 9, No. 31, 1987, p. 63.

501. Gaur, R. D. and Semwal, J. K. "Exploitation and threat to some high altitude plants in Garhwal Himalaya". In Assessment of Threatened Plants of India. B. Si., Calcutta, 1984, pp. 37-39.

502. Gaur, R. D. and Semwal, J. K. "Some little known wild edible of Garhwal Himalaya". *Man and Environment,* Vol. 7, 1983, pp. 161-165.

503. Gaur, R. D. and Tiwari, J. K. "Some little known medicinal plants of Garhwal Himalaya: An ethnobotanical study". In Medicinal and Poisonous Plants of the Tropicsedited by Leewenberg, Netherland, 1987, pp. 139-192.

504. Gaur, R.D., Bhatt, K. C. & Tiwari, J. K. "An ethnobotanical study of Uttar Pradesh Himalaya in relation to veterinary

medicines". *Journal of Indian Botanical Society*, Vol. 72, 1992, 139-144.

505. Gaur, R.D., Bisht, M. K. and Bhatt, K. C. "A note on medicinal and other uses of some animal in Garhwal Himalaya: An ethnozoological perspective". *Man in India*, Vol. 68, No. 2&3, 1988, pp. 292-297.

506. Gaur, R. D., Purohit, V. P. & Silas, R. A. "Eunymus tingens Wall. (Celastraceae) –A tree of multieconomic folk utility in Raath region (Garhwal Himalaya)". *Bulletin of the Botanical Survey of India*, Vol. 28, 1986, pp. 146-148.

507. Gaur, R. D., Semwal, J. K. and Sharma, M. P. "Ethnotoxic plants of Garhwal Hills". *Eastern Anthropologist*, Vol. 33, 1980, pp. 159-163.

508. Gaur, Vaidya Banwari Lal "Understanding Ayurveda". Jaipur, Publication Scheme, 2002, p. 246.

509. Gavali, Deepa and Sharma, Diwakar "Traditional knowledge and biodiversity conservation in Gujarat". *Indian Journal of Traditional Knowledge,* Vol. 3, No.1, 2004, pp. 51-58.

510. Geetha, S. G. Lakshmi & Ranjithakani, P. "Ethnobotanical review: wild fibre yielding plants of Kolli hills, Tamil Nadu". In Ethnobotany and Medicinal Plants of Indian Sub-continent, edited by J. K. Maheshwari, Jodhpur, India Scientific Publishers, 2000.

511. Geetha, S., Lakshmi, G. & Ranjithakani, P. "Ethno-veterinary medicinal plants of Kolli hills, Tamil Nadu". In Ethnobotany and Medicinal Plants of Indian Sub-continent, edited by J. K. Maheshwari, Jodhpur, India Scientific Publishers, 2000.

512. Genarjee, G., Srikanth, K. and Ramu, G. "Ethnozoological study in a tropical wildlife sanctuary of Eturunagaram in the Warangal district, Andhra Pradesh". *Indian Journal of Traditional Knowledge,* Vol. 9, No. 4, 2010, pp.710-704.

513. George, P. S. Satheesh, Tushar, K. V. and Balachandran, Indira "Medicinal Plants used by the Kaadar tribes of Sholayar forest, Thrissur district, Kerala". *Indian Journal of Traditional Knowledge,* Vol. 4, No. 2, 2005, pp. 159-163.

514. Gerson, S. "Ayurveda: ancient India healing art". Shaftsburg, England, Element, 1993.

515. Gharami, Ajay Kr. and Sharma, A. N. "An appraisal of traditional medicine and treatment among Nicobarese of Little Andaman". *Vanyajati*, Vol. 49, No. 1, 2001, pp. 5-10.

516. Ghatapanadi, S. R., Johnson, Nicky and Rajasab, A. H. "Documentation of Folk Knowledge on medicinal plants of Gulbarga district, Karnataka". *Indian Journal of Traditional Knowledge,* Vol. 10, No. 2, 2011, pp. 349-353.

517. Ghorband, Dnyaneshwar, Biradar, P. Sharad, D. "Traditional medicines knowledge in Dharmabad taluka of Nanded district, Maharashtra, India". *Indian Journal of Natural Products and Resources*, Vol. 2, No. 4, 2011, pp. 498-503.

518. Ghosal, S. "Tree in folklife". *Folklore*, Vol. 6, 1965, pp. 179-190.

519. Ghosal, Samit and Thakre, R. B. "Indigenous management of maritime resources: A study on marine fisher folk Kolis of the Raigarh district in Maharashtra". *Journal of Indian Anthropological Society,* Vol. 45 No. 2, 2010, pp. 123-141.

520. Ghosh, Abhik "Mythologies of the everyday: tribal health and medicine in Jharkhand". *Man in India*, Vol. 85, No. 3-4, 2005, pp. 209-220.

521. Ghosh, Abhik "Oraon worldviews and concepts of health and medicine". *Man in India*, Vol .76, No. 1, 1996, pp. 67-80.

522. Ghosh, Ashis "Ethno veterinary medicines from the tribal areas of Bankura and Medinipur districts, West Bengal". *Indian Indian Journal of Traditional Knowledge,* Vol. 1, No. 1, 2002, pp. 93-95.

523. Ghosh, Ashis "Herbal folk remedies of Bankura and Medinipur districts, West Bengal". *Indian Journal of Traditional Knowledge,* Vol. 2, No. 4, 2003, pp. 393-396.

524. Ghosh, Ashis, Maity, Sarathi & Maity, Malaty "Ethnomedicine in Bankura district, West Bengal". In Ethnobotany and Medicinal Plants of Indian Sub-continent, edited by J. K. Maheshwari, Jodhpur, India Scientific Publishers, 2000.

525. Ghosh, T. K., Mahato, A. K. & Sahu, S. C. "Some important medicinal plants used against dysentery by the tribals of

Chota Nagpur and Santhal Pargana (Bihar)". Proceedings of 67th Indian Science Congress Pt III (Abstract), 1980, p. 63.

526. Ghoshmaulik, S. K. and Karmohapatra, R. K. "Health situation of the Juands of Orissa". *South Asian Anthropologist,* Vol. 16, No. 2, 1995, pp. 79-83.

527. Girach, R. D. "Ethnobotanical notes on some Plants of Mahendragiri Hills, Orissa". *Ethnobotany*, Vol .13, No. 1-2, 2001, pp. 80-83.

528. Girach, R. D. and Aminuddin "Ethnomedicinal Uses of Plants among the tribals of Singbhum district, Bihar, India". *Ethnobotany*, Vol.7, No. 1-2, 1995, pp. 103-107.

529. Girach, R. D., Aminuddin and Brahmam, M. "Observations on Ethnomedicinal Plants of Bhadrak district, Orissa, India". *Ethnobotany*, Vol . 9, No. 1-2, 1997, pp. 44-46.

530. Girach, R. D., Singh, S, Brahman, M., Misra, M. K. "Traditional treatment of skin diseases in Bhadrak district, Orissa". In Ethnobotany and medicinal plant of Indian subcontinent, edited by J. K. Maheshwari, Saujanya Books, Jodhpur, 2003, p. 672.

531. Gnanambal, K. "The religious beliefs of the Urali". *Bulletin of the Department of Anthropology*, Vol. 4, No. 2, 1955.

532. Godwa, M. "The story of Pan Chewing in India". Botanical Museum Leaflets Harward University Vol. 4, 1950, pp. 181-214.

533. Goel, A. K. and Bhattacharya, U. C. "A note on some plants found effective in treatment of jaundice (Hepatitis)". *Journal of Economic and Taxonomic Botany*, Vol. 2, 1981, pp. 157-159.

534. Goel, A. K. and Mudgal, V. "A Survey of medicinal plants used by the tribal of Santal Pargana (Bihar)". *Journal of Economic and Taxonomic Botany*, Vol. 12, 1988, pp. 329-335.

535. Goel, A. K., Sahoo, A. K. and Mudgal, V. "A contribution to the ethnobotany of Santal Paragana". Botanical Survey of India, Howrah, Calcutta, 1984.

536. Goel, A. K., Sahoo, A. K. and Mudgal, V. "Medico-ethnobotany of the Santal Pargana (Bihar), Stomach and

gastric disorders". *The Eastern Anthropologist*, Vol. 40, No. 2, 1987, pp. 162-168.

537. Gogoi, P. and Boissya, C. L. "Informations about a few herbals medicines used by the people of Assam (India) against jaundice". *Himalayan Research Development,* Vol. 2, 1984, pp. 41-44.

538. Gopal, K. Rani "Tribals and their health status". A.P.H. Publishing, New Delhi, 1996, p. 135.

539. Gorband, Dnyaneshwar P. and Biradar, Sharad, P. "Folk medicine used by the tribes of Kinwat forest of Nanded district, Maharashtra, India". *Indian Journal of Natural Products and Resources,* Vol. 3, No. 1, 2012, pp. 118-122.

540. Goswami, Anvita, Dixit, Vinod K. and Srivastava, B. K. "Antimalarial trails on herbal extracts. I. clerodendron infortunatum L.". *Bionature*, Vol. 18, No. 2, 1998, pp. 45-49.

541. Goswami, Monali, Dash, Bijayalaxmi and Dash, N. C. "Traditional method of reproductive health care practices and fertility control among the Bhumja tribe of Baleswar, Orissa". *Studies on Ethno-medicine*, Vol. 5, No. 1, 2011, pp. 51-55.

542. Goswami, P. and Dutta, A. M. "Some folklore medicines of cardiac importance". *Ancient Science of Life*, Vol. 2, 1983, pp. 233-235.

543. Goswami, Pranjiv, Soki, Dudam and Jaishi, Ahju "Traditional healthcare practices among the Tagin tribe of Arunachal pradesh". *Indian Journal of Traditional Knowledge,* Vol. 8, No. 1, 2009, pp. 93-95.

544. Gould H. A. "Modern medicine and folk cognition in rural India". *Human organization*, Vol. 25, 1965, pp. 122-125.

545. Gould, H. A. "The Implications of technological change for folk and scientific medicine". *American Anthropologist,* Vol. 59, 1957, pp. 507-516.

546. Gould, Harold A. "Modern Medicine and Folk Cognition in Rural India". In The Cross-Cultural Approach to Health Behaviour, edited by L. Riddick Lynch, Cranbury, New Jercy, Associated University Presses, 1969, pp. 316-336.

547. Gound, P Saiprasad and Pullaiah, T. "Folk veterinary

medicine of Kurnool district, Andhra Pradesh". *Ethnobotany*, Vol. 8, No. 1-2, 1996, pp. 71-74.

548. Govil, J. N. (ed.) "Current concepts of multidiscipline approach to the medicinal plants (2 Vols.)". New Delhi, Today and Tomorrow's Printers, 1998, p. 444.

549. Greenhalgh, Trisha "Drug prescription and self-medication in India: an exploratory study". *Social Science and Medicine*, Vol. 25, No. 3, 1987, pp. 307-318.

550. Griffith, W. G. "A visit to the Mismee hills in Assam". *Journal of Asiatic Society Bengal*, Vol. 6, 1837, pp. 325-341.

551. Grover, N. "Man and plants against pain". *Economic Botany* Vol. 19, 1965, pp. 99-112.

552. Guha, Anima "Folk medicine of the Bodo-Kacharis-A plains tribe of Assam". In Tribal health: Socio-cultural dimensions, edited by Buddhadeb Chaudhuri, New Delhi, Inter-India publications, 1986, pp. 191-200.

553. Guha, P. "Betal leaf: The neglected green gold of India". *Journal of Human Ecology*, Vol. 19, No. 2, 2006, pp. 87-93.

554. Guite, Nemthianngai and Acharya, Sanghmitra S. "Indigenous medicinal substances and health care: A study among paite tribe of Manipur, India". *Studies of Tribes and Tribals*, Vol. 4, No. 2, 2006, pp. 99-108.

555. Guna, B. S. "Medicine Man of the Abor Hills". *The Times of India*, 25 Oct. 1959.

556. Gupta, B. L. "Forest Flora of Chakrata Dehra Dun and Saharanpur Forest Division". United Provinces, Calcutta, 1928.

557. Gupta, Beni, "Magical beliefs and superstitions". Delhi, Sundeep Prakashan, 1979.

558. Gupta, Brahmananda "Evolution of Ayurveda through the ages". In History of medicine in India: the Medical encounter, edited by Chittabrata Palit and Achintya Dutta, Delhi, Kalpaz Publications, 2005, pp. 207-218.

559. Gupta, K. R. L. "Hindu-anatomy, physiology, therapeutics, history of medicine and practice of physic". Delhi, Sri Satguru, 1986, p. 209.

560. Gupta, Kaviraj Russick Lal "Ayurvedic System of Pathology: roga nidanam". Delhi, Vedic Books, 2006, p. 294.

561. Gupta, M. L., Gupta, T. K. and Bhargava, K. P. "A study of antifertility effect of some indigenous drugs". *Journal of Research in Indian Medicine*, Vol. 6, No.2, 1971, pp. 6-116.

562. Gupta, Mradu, Biswas, Tuhin Kant and Saha, Shyamali "Therapeutic utilization of secretory products of some Indian medicinal plants-a review". *Indian Journal of Traditional Knowledge,* Vol. 5, No. 4, 2006, pp. 569-575.

563. Gupta, R. "Medicinal plants of West Himalaya". *Journal of Agric. Trop. Bot. Applied,* Vol. 9, 1962, pp. 1-54.

564. Gupta, R. "Plants in folk-medicine of the Himalayas". In Glimpses of Indian Ethnobotany, edited by S. K. Jain, 1981, pp. 83-90.

565. Gupta, R. K. "Some useful and medicinal plants of Garhwal Himalaya: An ethnobotanical study". In Medicinal and Poisonous Plants of the Tropics edited by Leewenberg, 1960, pp: 139-142.

566. Gupta, R. K. "Some useful and medicinal plants of Nainital district in the Kumaun Himalaya". *Indian Forester*, Vol. 57, 1960, pp. 309-324.

567. Gupta, R. K. "Some useful and medicinal plants of Nainital in Kumaun Himalaya". *Journal of Bombay Natural History Society*, Vol. 68, No. 3, 1960, pp. 791-803.

568. Gupta, Rakhi, Vairale, M. G. and Deshmukh, R.R. "Ethnomedicinal uses of some plants used by Gond tribe of Bhandara district, Maharashtra". *Indian Journal of Traditional Knowledge,* Vol. 9, No. 4, 2010, pp. 713-717.

569. Gupta, S. P. "An Appraisal of chotanagpur tribal pharmacooeia". *Bulletin of the Bihar Tribal Research Institute*, Vol. 5, No. 2, 1963, pp. 1-18.

570. Gupta, S. P. "Folk-lore about plants with reference to Munda culture". In Glimpses of Indian ethnobatany, edited by S. K. Jain, 1981, pp. 119-207.

571. Gupta, S. P. "Native medicinal uses of plants by the Asurs of Netarhat plateau (Bihar)". In Glimpses of Indian Ethnobotany edited by S. K. Jain, 1981, pp. 218-231.

572. Gupta, S. P. "Tribal concept of health disease and remedy". In Tribal health: Socio-Cultural dimentions, edited by Buddhadeb Chaudhuri, New Delhi, Inter India, 1986, pp. 161-166.

573. Gupta, S. P. "Tribal health and medicine: a key note address". In Education and health problems in tribal development: a study of National integration edited by Kanchan Roy, Concept Publishing House, 1989, pp. 81-88.

574. Gupta, S. P. "Tribes of Chotanagpur plateau. An Ethnonutritional and pharmacological cross-section". Ranchi, Bihar Tribal Welfare Research Institute, 1969.

575. Gupta, Satya Prakash "Chotanagpur tribes: Their health and herbal medicines". *South Asian Anthropologist*, Vol. 9, No. 1, 1988, pp. 25-35.

576. Gupta, Shakti M. "Plant myths and traditions in India". New Delhi, Munshiram Manoharlal, 1991, p. 123.

577. Gupta, Stutee, Porwal, M. C. and Roy, P. S. "Indigenous knowledge on some medicinal plants among the Nicobari tribe of Car Nicobar Island". *Indian Journal of Traditional Knowledge,* Vol. 3, No. 3, 2004, pp. 287-293.

578. Gupta, Vishal "Plants used in folklore medicine by Bangnis of east Kameng, Arunachal Pradesh". *Indian Journal of Natural Products and Resources*, Vol. 5, No. 1, 2006, pp. 52-59.

579. Gurmet, Padma and others "Some traditional medicinal plants of Khardungla and Changla (Ladakh) used in Amchi medicine". *Bulletin of Medico-Ethno-Botanical Research,* Vol. 19, No. 3-4, 1998, pp. 93-101.

580. Gurukkal, R. Rajeev "The art of fighting and healing". *Discover India,* Vol. 13, no. 6, 2000, pp. 20-21.

581. Gurumayum, S. D. and Choudhury, M. "Fishing methods in the rivers of northern India". *Indian Journal of Traditional Knowledge,* Vol. 8, No. 2, 2009, pp. 237-241.

582. Habib, S. Irfan, and Raina, Dhruv "Reinventing traditional medicine: Method, institutional change, and the manufacture of drugs and medication in late colonial India". In Asian medicine and globalization edited by Joseph S. Alter, Philadelphia, University of Pennsylvania Press, 2005, pp. 67-77.

583. Haekel, J. "Some aspects of the social life of the Bhilala in Central India". *Ethnology*, Vol. 2, No. 2, 1963, pp. 190-206.

584. Hajra, P. K. "Nature conservation in Khasi folk beliefs and taboos". In Glimpses of Indian Ethnobotany edited by S.K. Jain, New Delhi, Oxford & IBH, 1980, pp. 149-152.

585. Hajra, P. K. "Plants in magico-religious beliefs and in sankrit literature". In A manual of ethnobotany, edited by S. K. Jain, Scientific Publishers, Jodhpur, 1995, pp. 98-103.

586. Hajra, P. K. "Some important medicinal plants from Kameng district, Arunachal Pradesh". *Bulletin of Meghalaya Science Society*, Vol. 2. 1977, pp. 16-20.

587. Haldar, Asesh Kumar "The Sauria Paharia: A study of Ethno-Medical system". Midnapur, Rarh Samskriti Sangrahalaya, 1998, p. 96.

588. Haldar, J. R. "Medical science in Pali literature". Calcutta, Indian Museum, 1977, p. 72.

589. Hall, O. "Sociological Research in the field of medicine: progress and prospects". *American sociological Review*, Vol. 16, pp. 639-44.

590. Halliburton, Murphy "Resistance or inaction?: Protecting ayurvedic medical knowledge and problems". *American Ethnologist*, Vol. 38, No. 1, 2011, pp. 86-101.

591. Halliburton, Murphy "The importance of a pleasant process of treatment: Lessons from healing from South India". Culture, Medicine and Psychiatry, Vol. 27, 2003, pp. 161-186.

592. Hardiman, David "Missionaries and their medicine: a Christian modernity for tribal India". Manchester University Press, Manchester, 2008, p. 261.

593. Hardiman, David and Raje, Gauri "Practices of healing in tribal Gujarat". *Economic and Political Weekly*, Vol. 43, No. 9, 2008, pp. 43-50.

594. Harilal, M. S. "Commercialising traditional medicine: Ayurvedic manufacturing in Kerala". *Economic and Political Weekly,* Vol. 44, No. 16, 2009, pp. 44-51.

595. Harsha, V. H., Hebber, S.S., Shripathi, V., Hedge, G.R., "Ethnomedicobotany of Uttara Kannada District in

Karnataka, India-plants in treatment of skin diseases". *Journal of Ethnopharmacology*, Vol. 84, No. 1, 2003, pp. 37-40.

596. Harsha, V. H., Shripathi, V. and Hegde, G. R. "Ethnoveterinary practices in Uttara Kannada district of Karnataka". *Indian Journal of Traditional Knowledge,* Vol. 4, No. 3, 2005, pp. 253-258.

597. Hartmann, Franz "Occult science in medicine". New York, Samuel Weiser, 1975, p. 100.

598. Hasan, Amir "Role of the Bharra among the Tharu: A tribe of mongoloid origin" *Folklore*, Vol. 33, No. 3, 1992, pp. 66-69.

599. Hasan, Khwaja A. "The Hindu dietary practices and culinary rituals in a North Indian village: an ethnomedical and structural analysis". *Ethnomedicin / Ethnomedicine*, Vol. 1, 1971, pp. 43-70.

600. Hasnain, N. "Tribal India Today". Harnam Publications, New Delhi, 1990.

601. Hassan, I. "Some folk uses of peganum harmala in India and Pakistan". *Economic Botany*. Vol. 21, 1967, pp. 284.

602. Hassen, A. K. "Drinks, drugs and disease in a north Indian village". *Eastern Anthropology*, Vol. 17, 1964, pp. 1-9.

603. Hatfield, Gabrielle "Encyclopedia of Folk Medicine: Old World and New world Traditions". Gurgaon, Shubhi Publication, 2004. p. 392.

604. Hebbar, S. S., Harsha, V. H., Shripathi, V. and Hedge, G.R. "Ethnomedicine of Dharwad district in Karnataka, India-plant used in oral health care". *Journal of Ethnopharmacology*, Vol. 94, 2004, pp. 261-266.

605. Helmholtz, Hermann Von "Science and culture: popular and philosophical essays". Chicago, University of Chicago Press, 1995, p. 418.

606. Hema, E. S., Sivadasan, M. and Kumar, N. Anil "Studies on edible species of amaranthaceae and araceae used by Kuruma and Paniya tribes in Wayanad district, Kerala, India". *Ethnobotany*, Vol .18, No. 1-2, 2006, pp. 122-126.

607. Hemadri, K. and Raj, P. V., Rao, S. S. & Sarma, C. R. R. "Folklore claims from Andhra Pradesh-1". *Journal of*

Science Research Plant Medicine, Vol. 1, No.2, 1980, pp. 37-49.

608. Hemadri, K., Sarma, C. R. R. & Rao, S. S. "Medicinal plant wealth of Andhra Pradesh-Part 1". *Ancient Science of Life*, Vol. 6, 1987, pp. 167-186.

609. Hemadri, Koppula "Jaundice: Tribal medicine". *Ancient Science of Life*, Vol. 3, No.4, 1981, pp. 209-212.

610. Hemadri, Koppula "Medico-botanical exploration of Phulbani and Koraput district of Orissa". Central Council for Research in Ayurveda and Siddha". New Delhi, 1991.

611. Hemadri, Koppula "Rheumatism: tribal medicine". *Ancient Science of Life*, Vol. 1, No. 2, 1981, pp. 117—120.

612. Hemadri, Koppula and Rao, Swahari Sasibhushana "Folk Medicine of Bastar". *Ethnobotany*, Vol .1, No. 1-2, 1989, pp. 61-66.

613. Hemadri, Koppula and Rao, Swahari Sasibhushana "Leucorrhoea and menorrhagia: tribal medicine". *Ancient Science of Life,* Vol. 3, No. 1, 1983, pp.40-41.

614. Hembrom, Peter Paul "Contact therapy practised by Mundas of Chotanagpur (Bihar)". *Ethnobotany*, Vol. 3, No. 1&2, 1991, pp. 36-39.

615. Hembrom, Peter Paul "Tribal medicine in Chotanagpur and Santhal Parganas of Bihar, India". *Ethnobotany*, Vol. 3, No. 1&2, 1991, pp. 97-99.

616. Hembrom, Peter Paul and Goel, Anil K "Horopathy: ethnomedicine of Mundas". *Ethnobotany*, Vol. 17, No. 1-2, 2005, pp. 89-95.

617. Hemlata, Oinam and Kumari, Pebam Krishna "Health care practices among tribes of Manipur". In Tribal health and medicines, edited by A. K. Kalla and P. C. Joshi, New Delhi: Concept Publishing Co., 2004, pp. 276-282.

618. Henry, Edward O. "A North Indian Healer and the sources of his power". In Main currents in Indian sociology, edited by Giriraj Gupta, Vol. 4, New Delhi: Vikas Publishing House Pvt. Ltd. pp. 286-307, 1981.

619. Henry, Edward O. "A North Indian Healer and the Sources of His Power". *Social Science and Medicine*, Vol. 11, No. 15, 1997, pp. 309-317.

620. Heredia, Rudolf C. "Social medicine for holistic health: An alternative response to present crisis". *Economic and Political Weekly*, Vol. 25, No. 48-49, 1990, pp. 2673-80.

621. Hoernle, A. F. Rudolf "Studies in the medicine of ancient India: osteology or the bones of the human body". New Delhi, Concept, 1994, p. 252.

622. Hoernle, A. F. Rudolf "Studies in the medicine of ancient India". Part I, Oxford 1907.

623. Hoff, Wilbur and Maseko, D., Nhlavana. "Nurses and traditional healers join hands". *World Health Forum*, Vol. 7, No. 4, 1986.

624. Hosagoudar, V. B. and A. N. Henry "Ethnobotany of Kadars, Malasars and Muthuvans of Anamalais in Coimbatore district, Tamil Nadu, India". In Ethnobotany and Medicinal Plants of Indian Sub-continent, edited by J. K. Maheshwari, Jodhpur, India Scientific Publishers, 2000.

625. Hosagoudar, V. B. and Henry, A. N. "Ethnobotany of tribes Irular, Kurumban and Paniyan of Nilgiris in Tamil Nadu, Southern India". In Ethnobotany and Medicinal Plants of Indian Sub-continent, edited by J. K. Maheshwari, Jodhpur, India Scientific Publishers, 2000.

626. Hosagoudar, V.B. and Henry, A. N. "Ethnobotany of Soligas in Biligiri Rangana, Karnataka, Southern India". In Ethnobotany and Medicinal Plants of Indian Sub-continent, edited by J. K. Maheshwari, Jodhpur, India Scientific Publishers, 2000.

627. Hrudayanath Thatoi and Rout, Srustidhar "Medicinal Plants Ethnomedicine and Biotechnological Potential". 2011, p. 407.

628. Huffman, M. A. and Seifu, M. "The use of medicinal plants by primates: A missing link?". *Primates*, Vol. 30, No. 1, 1989, pp. 51-63.

629. Hugh and Gantzer, Colleen "Healing waters". *Discover India*, Vol. 13, No. 8, 2000, 2000, pp. 10-13.

630. Hughes Charles C, "Ethnomedicine". In International Encyclopedia of the social sciences (Vol. 10) edited by David L. Sills, New York, Free Press/ Macmillan, 1968, pp. 87-93.

631. Huidrom, B. K. Singh "Plants used in medico-sexual purposes by Meitei community in Manipur state, India". In Ethnobotany and Medicinal Plants of Indian Sub-continent, edited by J. K. Maheshwari, Jodhpur, India Scientific Publishers, 2000.

632. Hussain and Ali, Arif. "Relevance of ethnomedicine". *Man and Life,* Vol. 18, No.1and 2, Calcutta, 1992.

633. Hussian, Syed Khaza, M. "Medicine among the Gonds, Kolams and Chenchus". *Man in India*, Vol. 30, 1950, pp. 23-31.

634. Hyma, A., Ramesh, A. and Subhadra, N. L. "Development of a rural community health care model based on Indian indigenous system of medicine". *Ancient Science of Life,* Vol. 8, No. 2, 1988, pp. 138-166.

635. Hynniewia, S.R. and Kumar, Y. "The lesser-known medicine Ka Dawai Niangsohpet of the Khasis in Meghalaya, Northeast India". *Indian Journal of Traditional Knowledge,* Vol. 9, No. 3, 2009, pp. 475-479.

636. Hynniewta, S. R. and Kumar, Yogendra "Herbal remedies among the Khasi traditional healers and village folks in Meghalaya". *Indian Journal of Traditional Knowledge,* Vol. 7, No. 4, 2008, pp. 581-586.

637. Ibata, Atsuko "Bon medicine among monpas in Western Arunachal". In Tribal health and medicines, edited by A. K. Kalla and P. C. Joshi, New Delhi: Concept Publishing Co., 2004, p.p. 318-342.

638. Ignacimuthu S, Ayyanar M, Sivaraman S. "Ethnobotanical investigations among tribes in Madurai District of Tamil Nadu (India)". *Journal of Ethnobiology and Ethnomedicine*, Vol. 2, No. 25, 2006. (Bio Med Central Full Text)

639. Imam, S., Hussain, S. J., Gupta, V. C. and Hussain, M. "Folk herbal drugs for snakebites from Andhra Pradesh Forests". In International Seminar on Traditional Medicine, Calcutta, Abstr. No. 144, 1992.

640. International Indigenous Commission, "Indigenous Peoples, Traditional Knowledge and Management Practices: a report prepared for the United Nations Conference on Environment and Development". 1991.

641. Islam M. "Ethnobotany of certain underground parts of plants of north-eastern region, India". In Ethnobotany and Medicinal Plants of Indian Sub-continent, edited by J. K. Maheshwari, Jodhpur, India Scientific Publishers, 2000.

642. Issar, R. K. "A note on the botanical source of a snake bite anti-dote drug 'Nagdaun'". *Journal of Research in Indian Medicine*, Vol. 10, No. 4, 1975, p. 171.

643. Issar, R. K. "Traditionally important medicinal plants and folk-lore of Uttarakhand Himalaya for animal treatment". *Journal of Science Research Plant Medicine*, Vol. 2, 1981, pp. 61-66.

644. Jacob, Miaron O., Farah, Kassim O. and Ekaya, Wellington N. "Indigenous knowledge: The basis of the Maasai ethnoveterinary diagnostic skills". *Journal of Human Ecology*, Vol. 16, No. 1, 2004, pp. 43-48.

645. Jadeja, B. A. "Plants used by the tribe Rabari in Barda Hills of Gujrat". *Ethnobotany*, Vol.11, No. 1-2, 1999, pp. 42-46.

646. Jadeja, B. A., Odedra, N. K. and Odedra, K. R. "Herbal remedies used for haemorrhoids by tribals of Saurashtra, Gujarat". *Indian Journal of Traditional Knowledge,* Vol. 5, No. 3, 2006, pp. 348-352.

647. Jadeja, B. A., Odedra, N. K. and Solanki, K. M."Indigenous animal healthcare practices in district Porbandar, Gujarat". *Indian Journal of Traditional Knowledge,* Vol. 5, No. 2, 2006, pp. 253-258.

648. Jadhav Dinesh "Ethnomedicinal plants used by Bhil tribe of Bidbod, M.P.". *Indian Journl of Traditional Knowledge*, Vol. 5, No. 2, 2006, pp. 263-267.

649. Jadhav Dinesh "Ethnomedicinal plants used for curing skin affictions by Bhil tribe of Ratlam district, Madhya Pradesh". *Journal of Economic and Taxonomic Botany,* Vol. 30, Supp., pp. 124-127.

650. Jadhav Dinesh "Plant sources used for the treatment of types of fevers by Bhil tribe of Ratlam district, Madhya Pradesh". *Journal of Economic and Taxonomic Botany*, Vol. 30, No. 4, pp. 909-911.

651. Jadhav, Dinesh "Amulets and other plant wearings believed

to be contact therapy among tribals of Ratlam district (MP) India". *Ethnobotany*, Vol. 20, No. 1&2, 2008, pp. 144-146.

652. Jadhav, Dinesh "Ethno-gynaecological uses of plants by Bhil tribe of Ratlam district (MP)". *Ethnobotany*, Vol .22, No. 1-2, 2010, pp. 138-141.

653. Jadhav, Dinesh "Ethno-Medicinal Survey of Maalgamdi in Ujjain district, Madhya Pradesh, India". *Ethnobotany*, Vol.18, No. 1-2, 2006, pp. 157-159.

654. Jadhav, Dinesh "Ethnomedicinal survey of tribal inhabited localities of Ratlam district (MP) in the light of 'doctrine of signatures'". *Ethnobotany*, Vol. 23, No. 1&2, 2011, pp. 121-124.

655. Jaggi, O. P. "Ayurveda: Indian system of medicine". Delhi: Atma Ram & Sons, 1981, p. 256.

656. Jaggi, O. P. "Folk medicine". Delhi, Atma Ram & Sons, 1982, p. 228.

657. Jaggi, O. P. "Yogic and tantric medicine". Delhi, Atma Ram, 1979, p. 206.

658. Jagtap, S. D. and others "Antimicrobial activity of some crude herbal drugs used for skin diseases by Pawra tribes of Nandurbar district". *Indian Journal of Natural Products and Resources,* Vol. 1, No. 2, 2010, pp. 216-220.

659. Jain, A, Katewa, S.S., Galav, P.K., Nag, A. "Unrecorded ethnomedicinal uses of biodiversity from Tadgarh-Raoli Wildlife Sanctuary, Rajasthan, India". *Acta Botanica Indica,* Vol. 29, No. 3, 2007, pp. 337-344.

660. Jain, Alka, Roshnibala, S. and Kanjilal, P. B. "Aquatic/semi-aquatic plants used in herbal remedies in the wetlands of Manipur, Northeastern India". *Indian Journal of Traditional Knowledge,* Vol. 6, No. 2, 2007, pp. 346-351.

661. Jain, Anita, Katewa, S .S. and Galav, Praveen "Some therapeutic uses of biodiversity among the tribals of Rajasthan". *Indian Journal of Traditional Knowledge,* Vol. 7, No. 2, 2008, pp. 256-262.

662. Jain, Anita, Katewa, S.S. and Galav, P.K. "Some phytotherapeutic claims by tribals of southern Rajasthan". *Indian Journal of Traditional Knowledge,* Vol. 4, No. 3, 2005, pp. 291-297.

663. Jain, Anita, Katewa, S. S. and Sharma, S. K. "Snakelore and indigenous snakebite remedies practiced by some tribals of Rajasthan". *Indian Journal of Traditional Knowledge,* Vol. 10, No. 2, 2011, pp. 258-268.

664. Jain, Ashok K. "Folklore claims on snakebite among some tribal communities of central India: Kadel, Chitralekha". *Indian Journal of Traditional Knowledge,* Vol. 7, No. 2, 2008, pp. 269-299.

665. Jain, Ashok K. and Patole, Santosh N. "Less-known medicinal uses of plants among some tribal and rural communities of Pachmari Forest (M.P.)". *Ethnobotany,* Vol.13, No. 1-2, 2001, pp. 96-100.

666. Jain, Ashok K., Vairale, Mohan G. and Singh, Rajodeo "Folklore claims on some medicinal plants used by Bhil tribes of Guna district Madhya Pradesh". *Indian Journal of Traditional Knowledge,* Vol. 9, No. 1, 2010, pp. 105-107.

667. Jain, Ashok, K. and Tiwari, Preeti "Nutritional value of some traditional edible plants used by tribal communities during emergency with reference to Central India". *Indian Journal of Traditional Knowledge,* Vol. 11, No. 1, 2012, pp. 51-57.

668. Jain, C. M. and Bharathi, K. "Critical review of scientific validity of indigenous female contraceptive drugs described in ayurvedic literature". *Indian Journal of Traditional Knowledge,* Vol. 10, No. 4, 2011, pp. 678-681.

669. Jain, M.K. and A.C. Dubey "A study of traditional medicines in the Saur tribe of Tikamgarh District, Madhya Pradesh". *Tribal Health Bulletin,* Vol. 6, No. 2, 2000, pp. 11-13.

670. Jain, S.C., Jain, R. and Singh, R. "Ethnobotanical survey of Sariska and Siliserh regions from Alwar district of Rajasthan, India". *Ethnobotanical Leafletts,* Vol. 13, 2009, pp. 171-188.

671. Jain, S.K. "Credibility of traditional knowledge- the criterion of multilocational and multiethnic use". *Indian Journal of Traditional Knbowledge,* Vol. 3, No. 2, 2004, pp. 137-153.

672. Jain, S.K. (ed.) "Ethnobiology in Human Welfare". Deep Publication, New Delhi, 1996.

673. Jain, S.K. "An indigenous water bottle". *Indian forester*, Vol. 90, No. 10, 1964, p. 109.

674. Jain, S.K. "Dictionary of Indian folk Medicine and Ethno botany: A reference manual of man-plant relatonships etc". New Delhi, Deep Publication, 1991, p. 311.

675. Jain, S.K. "Dynamism in Ethnobotany". *Ethnobotany*, Vol. 17, No. 1-2, 2005, pp. 20-23.

676. Jain, S.K. "Dynamism of Traditional Knowledge". *Indian Journal of Traditional Knowledge,* Vol. 4, No. 2, 2005, pp. 115-117.

677. Jain, S.K. "Ethnobotanical research unfolds new vistas of traditional medicine in India". 1st International Conference on Traditional Asian Medicine, Canberra, 1979.

678. Jain, S.K. "Ethnobotany and traditional medicine". Keynote address, Asian Conference on Traditional Asian Medicine, Bombay, March 6-9, 1983.

679. Jain, S.K. "Grasses and rural life". *Khadigramodyog*, Vol. 12, 1966, pp. 324-326.

680. Jain, S.K. "Indian plants in traditional Tibetan medicine". *Ethnobotany*, Vol.15, No. 1-2, 2003, pp. 136-140.

681. Jain, S.K. "Magico-religious beliefs about plants among the adivasis of Bastar". *Quarterly Journal of the Mythic Society,* Vol. 54, No. 3, 1963, pp. 73-94.

682. Jain, S.K. "Medicinal plant-lore of the tribals of the Bastar". *Economic Botany*, Vol. 19, 1965, pp. 236-250.

683. Jain, S.K. "Medicinal plants", New Delhi, National book trust, 1975.

684. Jain, S.K. "Native plant remedies for snake bite among adivasis of central India". *Indian medical Journal*, Vol. 57, 1963, pp. 307-369.

685. Jain, S.K. "Notable foreign medicinal uses for some plants of India tradition". *Indian Journal of Traditional Knowledge,* Vol. 2, No. 4, 2003, pp. 321-332.

686. Jain, S.K. "Observation on ethnobotany of the tribals of Central India". In Glimpses of Indian Ethnobotany, edited by S.K. Jain, 1981.

687. Jain, S. K. "Observations on ethnobotany of the tribals of

Madhya Pradesh". *Vanyajati*, Vol. 11, No. 4, 1963, pp. 177-183.

688. Jain, S.K. "On the prospects of some new or less well known medicinal plants resources". *Indian Medical Journal*, Vol. 59, 1965, pp. 270-272.

689. Jain, S.K. "Plant resources in tribal areas of Bastar". *Khadigramodyog,* Vol. 10, 1964, pp. 557-561, also in *Vanyajati*, Vol. 12, 1964. pp. 147-173.

690. Jain, S. K. "Plants in Indian medicine and folklore associated with healing of bones". *Indian Journal Orthopedics*, Vol.1, 1967, pp. 95-104.

691. Jain, S. K. "Plants used in medicine by the tribals of Madhya Pradesh". *Bulletin of Regional Research Laboratory, Jammu,* Vol. 1, 1963, pp. 126-128.

692. Jain, S.K. "Some magico-religious beliefs about plants among Adibasis of Orissa". *Adibasi*, Vol. 12, 1971, pp. 39-44.

693. Jain, S. K. "Some traditional and cultural aspects of Biodiversity". *Ethnobotany*, Vol. 12, No. 1&2, 2000, pp. 128-134.

694. Jain, S. K. "Studies in Indian ethnobotany: Less known uses of 50 common plants from tribal areas of Madhya Pradesh". Bulletin of the Botanical Survy of India, Vol. 5, 1963, pp. 223-226.

695. Jain, S. K. "Studies in Indian ethnobotany: Origin and utility of some vernaculal plant names". Proceedings of the National Academy of Sciences. Vol. 33 B, No. 4, 1963, pp. 525-530.

696. Jain, S. K. "Studies in Indian ethnobotany-II. Plant used in medicine by tribals of Madhya Pradesh". *Bulletin of Regional Research Laboratory, Jammu*, Vol.1, 1963, pp. 126-128.

697. Jain, S. K. "The role of botanist in folk-lore research". *Folklore*, Vol. 5, No. 4, 1964, pp. 145-150.

698. Jain, S.K. "Utilisation of medicinal plants from wild sources". In Cultivation and utilisation of medicinal and aromatic plants edited by Atal C. K., Jammu, RRL, CSIR, 1977, pp. 461-467.

699. Jain, S.K. "Wild plant foods of the tribals of Bastar (Madhya Pradesh)". Proceedings of the National Academy of Sciences, Vol. 30 B, No. 2, 1964, pp. 56-80.

700. Jain, S.K. and Borthakur, S. K. "Ethnobotany of the Mikirs of India". *Economic Botany*, Vol. 34, 1980, pp. 264-272.

701. Jain, S.K. and De, J. N. "Some less known plant foods among the tribals of Purulia (West Bengal)". *Science and Culture,* Vol. 30, 1964, pp. 285-286.

702. Jain, S.K. and Goel, A.K. "Some Indian plants in Tibetan traditional medicine-I". *Ethnobotany*, Vol. 17, No. 1-2, 2005, pp. 127-136.

703. Jain, S.K. and Pal, D.C. "Ethnobotanical research on less known medicinal plants in India". In Cultivation and utilization of medicinal plants, edited by Atal C. K. and B. M. Kapur, Jammu, RRL, CSIR, 1982, pp. 538-557.

704. Jain, S.K. and Saklani, Arbind "Observations on the Tons valley region in the Uttarkashi district of the North-West Himalaya India". Mountain Research Development, Vol. 11, No. 2, 1991, pp. 157-161.

705. Jain, S.K. and Sastry, A.R.K. "Plant resources in the Himalayas". In Proceedings of National seminar on resources, development and environment in the Himalaya region, Department of Science and Technology, Govt. of India, New Delhi, 1980, pp. 98-107.

706. Jain, S. K. and Sharma, P. P. "A review of the parallel or unique indigenous uses of twenty-five plants in India and some African countries". *Ethnobotany*, Vol. 12, No. 1-2, 2000, pp. 51-55.

707. Jain, S.K. and Srivastava, Sumita "Some folk herbal medicines for possible use in veterinary practices". *Indian Journal of Traditional Knowledge,* Vol. 2, No. 2, 2003, pp. 118-125.

708. Jain, S.K. and Srivastava, Sumita "Traditional uses of some Indian plants among islanders of the Indian Ocean". *Indian Journal of Traditional Knowledge,* Vol. 4, No. 4, 2005, pp. 345-357.

709. Jain, S.K. and Tarafdar, C.R. "Studies in Indian ethnobotany-native plant remedies for snake-bite the

adibasis of central India". *Indian Medical Journal*, Vol. 57, 1963, pp. 307-309.

710. Jain, S.K. and Tarafder, C.R. "Medicinal plant lore of the Santals: A revival of P. O. Boddings work". *Economic Botany*, Vol. 24, 1970, pp. 270-278.

711. Jain, S.K., "Medicinal plant lores of the tribals of Bastar". *Economic Botany*, Vol. 19, No. 3, 1965, pp. 236-250.

712. Jain, S. K., "Role of folk-beliefs and practices in promoting health and combating diseases". Paper present at the 1st International Seminar of Unani Medicine, New Delhi, Feb., 13-15, 1987.

713. Jain, S. K., Banerjee, D. K. and Pal, D. C. "Medicinal plants among certain Adivasis in India". *Bulletin of Botanical Survey of India*, Vol. 15, No. 1 & 2, 1973, p. 85.

714. Jain, S. K., Hanfi, M. I. and Tarafdar, C. R. "Bauhinia vahlii-A multipurpose plants in tribal areas", *Vanyajati,* Vol. 21, No. 4, 1973, pp. 106-108.

715. Jain, S. K., Ranjan, Vinay and Sikarwar, R. L. S. "Botanical distribution of psychoactive plants of India". *Ethnobotany*, Vol. 6, No. 1-2, 1994, pp. 65-75.

716. Jain, S. K., Sinha, B. K. and Gupta, R. C. "Notable plants in ethnomedicine of India". New Delhi, Deep Publications, 1991, p. 219.

717. Jain, S. K., Sinha, B. K. and Saklani, Arvind "Some intresting medicinal plants known among several tribal societies of India". *Ethnobotany*, Vol. 1, No. 1&2, 1989, pp. 89-100.

718. Jain, S. P. "Ethno-medico-botanical survey of Chaibasa, Singhbhum district, Bihar". In Ethnobotany and Medicinal plants of Indian Sub-continent, edited by J. K. Maheshwari, Jodhpur, India Scientific Publishers, 2000.

719. Jain, S. P. "Medico-ethno-botanical survey of Dhar district, Madhya Pradesh". *Journal of Non-Timber Forest Products,* Vol. 11, No. 2, 2004, pp. 152-157.

720. Jain, S. P. and others "Hitherto unreported ethnomedicinal uses of plants of Betul district of Madhya Pradesh". *Indian Journal of Traditional Knowledge,* Vol. 9, No. 3, 2010, pp. 522-525.

721. Jain, S. P. and Singh, J. "Traditional medicinal practices among the tribal people of Raigarh (Chhattisgarh) India". *Indian Journal of Natural Products and resources,* Vol. 1, No. 1, 2010, pp. 109-115.

722. Jain, S. P., Srivastava, Sarika and Singh, J. "Traditional phytotherapy of Balaghat district, Madhya Pradesh, India". *Indian Journal of Traditional Knbowledge*. Vol. 10, No. 2, 2011, pp. 334-338.

723. Jain, Shashi Prabha "Gramin Samaj me Lok Chikitsa". New Delhi, Radha Publications, 2008, p. 181. [Hindi]

724. Jain, Sushil and Agarwal, Seema "Herbal medication: An alternative curative system among Bhils in Udaipur district". *The Anthropologist*, Vol. 5, No. 3, 2003, pp. 141-147.

725. Jamir, N. S. "Ethnobiology of Naga Tribe in Nagaland: I-medicinal herbs". *Ethnobotany*, Vol. 9, No. 1-2, 1997, pp. 101-104.

726. Jamir, N. S. "Fifty new or intresting Medicinal plants used by the Zeliangs of Nagaland: (India)". *Ethnobotany*, Vol.2, No. 1-2, 1990, pp. 11-18.

727. Jamir, N. S., Jungdan & Madhabi, S. "Traditional knowledge of medicinal plants µsed by the Yimchunger-Naga tribes in Nagaland". *Pleione*, Vol. 2, No. 2, 2008, pp. 223-228.

728. Jamir, N. S., Lanusunep & Konyak, C. H. Manwang "Some less known ethnomedicinal plants used by Angami-Naga tribes in Kohima district, Nagaland (India)". *Ethnobotany*, Vol. 23, No. 1-2, 2011, pp. 116-120.

729. Janardhanan, K. K. "Diseases of Major Medicinal plants". Delhi, Daya Publishing House, 2002, p. 189.

730. Janardhanan, K. K. "Malayalam Ergot poison and medicine" Thiruvanathapuram, State institute of languages, Kerala, 1995. p. 60.

731. Janardhanan, K. P. "An enumeration of the medicinal palnts of Khed Taluka Maharashtra State". *Bulletin of the Botanical Survey of India,* Vol. 5, 1963, pp. 363-374.

732. Jarvis, D. C. "Folk-medicine: A doctor guide to good health". London, W. H. Allen, 1960.

733. Jarvis, D. C., "Castor oil and corn oil". *Folk Medicine*, 1960, pp. 154-159.

734. Jarvis, D. C., "Some other uses of apple-cider vinegar in folk medicine". *Folk Medicine*, 1960, pp. 183-185.

735. Jarvis, D. C., "The usefulness of honey". *Folk Medicine*, 1960, pp.102-127.

736. Jayal, S. P. and Uniyal, M. P. "Medicnal plants of commercial and traditional importance in Bhilangana valley of Tehri Garhwal". *Nagarjun*, Vol. 10, No. 1, 1960, pp. 26-36.

737. Jayasundar, Rama "Ayurveda: A distinctive approach to health and disease". *Current Science*, Vol. 98, No. 7, 2010, pp. 908-914.

738. Jayasuriya, D.C. and Jayasuriya, Shanti "Legislation and regulation of traditional systems of medicine systems, practitioners and herbal products". In Traditional Medicine in Asia, edited by Ranjit Roy Chaudhury and Uton Muchtar Rafei, World Health Organization Regional Office for South-East Asia, New Delhi, 2001, pp. 159-182.

739. Jeetpuri "Vanvasi tatha unki Chamatkari Ausadhiya". *Vanyajati*, Vol. 18, No. 3, 1970, pp. 52-53. [Hindi]

740. Jeeva, S., Kiruba, S. and Mishra, B. P. "Weeds of Kanyakumari district and their value in rural life". *Indian Journal of Traditional Knowledge,* Vol. 5, No. 4, 2005, pp. 501-509.

741. Jeeva, S., Mishra, B. P. and Venugopal, N. "Traditional knowledge and biodiversity conservation in the sacred groves of Maghalaya". *Indian Journal of Traditional Knowledge,* Vol. 5, No. 4, 2006, pp. 563-568.

742. Jerath, B. K. "Synopsis of Social preventive medicine". Ludhiana, Man Mohan Jerath Publishers.

743. Jha, Amit "Traditional Indian medicine, with specific reference to Buddhist and tribal medicine". Research India Press, New Delhi, 2011, p. 372.

744. Jha, Amit, Jha, S., Suhag, V. "Ethnomedicinal plants of Lepchas of Dzongu area in Sikkim, India". *Crop Research,* Vol. 28, No. 1, 2 & 3, 2004, pp. 138-141.

745. Jha, R. R. "Plants used agains Cholera and Diarrhoea: Survey of Santal Medicine". Proceedings of Indian Science Congress, (abst.) 1989, p. 118.

746. Jha, R. R. "Sauaria Paharia Tribe and Plants: An analysis". *Ethnobotany*, Vol. 6, No. 1-2, 1994, pp. 87-93.

747. Jha, V. and Goel, Anil K. "Botanical Rosaries and Non-Flower Garlands in Folklore life of Mithila region: (North Bihar)". *Ethnobotany*, Vol.16, No. 1-2, 2004, pp. 27-32.

748. Jha, Vidyanath, Sunita Mishra, A.N. Kargupta and Abha Jha "Leaves and flowers utilized as supplementary vegetables in Darbhanga (North Bihar) and their ethnobotanical significance". In Ethnobotany and Medicinal plants of Indian Sub-continent, edited by J. K. Maheshwari, Jodhpur, India Scientific Publishers, 2000.

749. Jitha, T. J. "Mapping the life and works of Aiyappan". *Indian Anthropologist*". Vol. 40, No. 1, 2010, pp. 21-42.

750. Johari, Harish "Ancient Indian massage: traditional massage techniques based on the Ayurveda". New Delhi, Munshiram Manoharlal, 1984, p. 96.

751. John, D. "100 useful raw drugs of the Kani tribes of Trivendrum in Kerala". *Indian Journal of Crude Drug Research,* Vol. 22, No. 1, 1984, pp. 17-39.

752. Jones, David A. "Medical practice and tribal communities". In Health and disease in tribal societies". CIBA foundation symposium 49. New York, Elsevier excerpta Medica, 1977.

753. Jose, Priya and Sharma, B. V. "Utilisation of Indian systems of medicine: A study in Kaayaakalpa (Rejuvenation)". *Indian Journal of Traditional Knowledge,* Vol. 1, No. 1, 2002, pp. 11-16.

754. Jose, Priya and Sharma, B. V. "Utilisation of Indian systems of medicine: A study in Hyderabad, India". *South Asian Anthropologist,* Vol. 7, No. 2, 2007, 157-165.

755. Joseph, A. N. T. "Ethnozoology of reptiles in relation to health care among tribals in Madhya Pradesh". *Social Action,* Vol. 39, No. 4, 1989.

756. Joseph, J. and Kharkongor, P. "A preliminary ethnobotanical survey in the Khasi and Jaintia hills, Meghalaya". In Glimpses of Indian Ethno-botany, edited

by S. K. Jain, New Delhi, Oxford and IBH, 1980, pp. 115-123.

757. Joseph, Sarah "Indigenous social science project: Some political implications". *Economic and Political Weekly*, Vol. 26, No. 15, 1991, pp. 959-963.

758. Joseph, W. Eaton "Folk obstetrics and pediatrics meet the MD: A case study of social anthropology in medicine". In Patients, Physicians and Illness, edited by E. Gartly Jaco, New York, Free Press, 1958.

759. Joshi Pramila and Pande, P. C. "Ethnobotany of Bhotia tribe of Kumaun Himalaya". In Studies on Kumaun Himalaya edited by S. K. Sarma and N. C. Dhauondiyar, Indus Publishing Co., New Delhi. 1997, pp. 63-89.

760. Joshi, C. P. and Singh, B. B. "Indigenous agricultural knowledge on Kumaon hills of Uttaranchal". *Indian Journal of Traditional Knowledge,* Vol. 5, No. 1, 2006, pp. 19-24.

761. Joshi, D. N., Shah, B. C. L., & Suri, R. K. "Some medicinal plants of Rudranath Bugyal (Dist. Chamoli), U.P.". *Bulletin of Medico-Ethno Botanical Research,* Vol. 3, 1982, pp. 27-42.

762. Joshi, Devendra "Durlabh vanausadhiya se samradha hai Madhya Pradesh". A Journal of Democracy and development, Vol. 8, No. 2, 2008, pp. 15-17.

763. Joshi, G. C. "Ayurved anusandhan me vanaspatik sarvekshan evam papapalaya ki avashyakta-ek sujhava". *Sachitra Ayurved*, November, 1995, pp. 525-526. [Hindi]

764. Joshi, G. C. "New or little known plants from Kumoun Himalaya". *Journal of Economic and Taxonomic Botany,* Vol. 13, No. 2, 1989, pp. 347-348.

765. Joshi, G. C. "Notes on the vegetation types of inner Himalayan ranges of Kumaun Himalayaa with special reference to herbal resources". *Journal of Economic and Taxonomic Botany*, Vol. 17, No. 2, 1993, pp. 367-371.

766. Joshi, G. C. "Podophyllum hexandrum Royle: herbal drug a ray of hope for Cancers medicine". *Drugs Sachitra Ayurved*, July, 1993, pp. 55-56.

767. Joshi, G. C. and others "Botanical identification of new folk medicine for snakebite from Kamaun Himalaya". *Aryavaidyan*, Vol. 10, No. 2, 1996, pp. 114-115.

768. Joshi, G. C. and others "Resource survey of the pharmaceutically important plants of U.P. Himalaya". In Himalayan Biodiversity Conservation Strategies edited by U. Dhar, Gyanodya Prakashan, Nainital, 1993, pp. 279-291.

769. Joshi, G. C. and others "Uttarakhand Himalaya ke Shilajeet Sailkhando ke sansadhan serveksan per ek adhyan (in Hindi)". *Sachitra Ayurved*, July, 1993, pp. 33-34.

770. Joshi, G. C. and Pande, P. C. "Ethnobotany of Tarikhet block of Kumaun Himalaya". In Shikhar Salutation to the Himalaya edited by C. M. Agrwal, Indian Publishers & Distributors, Delhi, 2000, pp. 209-228.

771. Joshi, G. C. and Tewari, K. C. "Suggestion for medicinal plants cultivation". *Drugs Himalayan Research and Development*, Vol. 4, No. 2, 1985, pp. 43-46.

772. Joshi, G. C. and Tewari, V. P. "Danta rogon mai Uttrakhand ke ausadhi, Timoor (Zanthoxylum alatum) (in Hindi)". Drug Ayurved Vikas, November 1994.

773. Joshi, G. C. and Uniyal, M. R. "Folk medicinal importance of "Udsaleeb" Paeonia emodi Wall and its cultivation strategy from western Himalaya". *Drug Sachitra Ayurved,* August 1991, pp. 124-125.

774. Joshi, G. C. Tewari, V. P. & Joshi, P. "Geaster mammosum: A bactericidal fungus used in Himalayan folklore". *Journal of Ethnopharmacology*, Vol. 6, 1982, pp. 361-364.

775. Joshi, G. C., Pandey, N. K. & Uniyal, M. R. "Inventory of disappearing angiosperms of Kumaun and Garhwal Himalaya: causes and suggestions". *Journal of Economic and Taxonomic Botany*, Vol. 17, No. 2, 1993, pp. 421-432.

776. Joshi, G. C., Pandey, N. K., Tewari, K. C. & Tewari, R. N. "A preliminary synecological approach for the study of herbal wealth of high altitude Himalaya and their conservation strategy". *Bulletin of Medico-ethno-botanical Research,* Vol. 1-4, No. 6, 1991, pp. 98-102.

777. Joshi, G. C., Pandey, N. K., Tewari, V. P. & Tewari, K. C.

"Indigenous system of medicine and drug abuse". *Sachitra Ayurved*, July 1995, pp. 207-208.

778. Joshi, G. C., Tewari, K. C. & Pandey, G. "A review of indigenous system of medicine with special reference to herbal drugs". *Aryavaidyan*, Vol. 3, No. 3, 1992, pp. 173-179.

779. Joshi, G. C., Tewari, K. C. & Pandey, G. "A review of indigenous system of medicine with special reference to herbal drugs". *Aryavaidyan,* Vol. 3, No. 3, 1992, pp.173-179.

780. Joshi, G. C., Tewari, K. C. & Pandey, G. "Environmental pollution in relation to economic development causes and control". *Sachitra Ayurved*, January 1992, pp. 243-248.

781. Joshi, G. C., Tewari, K. C. & Tewari, V. P. "Alpine environs around Kamoun and Garwal in central Himalaya, India with special reference to herbal resources". *Bulletin of Medico-ethno-botanical Research,* Vol. 16, No. 3-4, 1995, pp. 114-122.

782. Joshi, G. C., Tewari, K. C., Pandey, N. K. & Pandey, G. "Dioscorea kumaonensis Kunth: A new source of anti hematic drug from Kumoun Himalaya and its conservation strategy". *Sachitra Ayurved*, March 1994, pp. 298-299.

783. Joshi, G. C., Tewari, K. C., Tewari, R. N. & Uniyal, M. R. "Conservation and large-scale cultivation strategy of Indian ginseng – Panax pseudoginseng Wall". *Indian Forester,* Vol. 117, No. 2, 1991, pp. 131-134.

784. Joshi, G. C., Tewari, N. K. & Tewari, D. N. "Depleting plant resources a case study from Kumaun Himalaya". *Journal of Economic and Taxonomic Botany,* Vol. 1, No. 2, 1987, pp. 13-16.

785. Joshi, G. C., Tewari, V. P. & Tewari, K. C. "Taxus baccata Linn. (Himalayan yew): an emerging anticancer plant drug". *Sachitra Ayurved*, February, 1995, pp. 611-612.

786. Joshi, Kalpana, Chavan, Preeti and Warude, Dnyaneshwar "Molecular markers in herbal drug technology". *Current Science*, Vol. 87, No. 2, 2004, pp. 159-165.

787. Joshi, M, C., Patel, M. B. & Mehta, P. J. "Some folk

medicines of Dangs, Gujrat state". *Bulletin of Medico-ethno-botanical Research,* Vol. 1, 1980, pp. 8-24.

788. Joshi, M. C. & Audichya, K. C. "Medicinal plants of Rajpopla forests of Gujrat State". *Bulletin of Medico-ethno-botanical Research,* Vol. 2, 1981, pp. 150-192.

789. Joshi, P. "An ethnobotanical study of Bhils-A preliminary survey". *Journal of Economic and Taxonomic Botany*, Vol. 3, 1982, pp. 257-266.

790. Joshi, P. "Ethnobotany of the Primitive tribes in Rajasthan". Printwell Jaipur, 1995.

791. Joshi, P. and Dhawan, V. "Swertia chirayita-an overview". *Current Science,* Vol. 89, No. 4, 2005, pp. 635-640.

792. Joshi, P. C. "The world of tribal healers". In Tribal health and medicines, edited by A. K. Kalla and P. C. Joshi, New Delhi: Concept Publishing Co., 2004, pp. 202-241.

793. Joshi, P. C. "Effective elements in the medical culture of Jaunsar-Bawar". *Research Proceedings*, Vol. 9, No. 1-2, 1982, pp. 35-49.

794. Joshi, P. C. "Ethnomedicine: explorations of some folk concepts in Jaunsar" Bawar Research Proceedings, Vol. 6, No. 1-2, 1978, Departmet of Anthropology, University of Delhi.

795. Joshi, P. C. "Issues in tribal health and medicines". In Tribal health and medicines, edited by A. K. Kalla and P. C. Joshi, New Delhi: Concept Publishing Co., 2004, pp. 403-444.

796. Joshi, P. C. "Medical anthropology: new areas of research in anthropology". Seminar on perspectives in Anthropological Researches in India: Planning for the future Researches and Methodologies, New Delhi: Delhi University. 27 September-1 October 1985.

797. Joshi, P. C. "Traditional medical system in Central Himalayas". *The Eastern Anthropologist*, Vol. 41, No. 1, 1988, pp. 77-86.

798. Joshi, P. C. "Traditional medical systems and the modern medical care planning for the underprivileged communities". Symposium on problems of development of underprivileged communities of the third World Countries, New Delhi, Department of Anthropology, Delhi University.

799. Joshi, P. C. "Tribal medicine in Indian context". *Vanyajati,* Vol. 42, No. 3, 1994, pp. 3-10.

800. Joshi, Prabhakar "Herbal Drugs in Tribal Rajasthan: from childbirth to childcare". *Ethnobotany,* Vol.1, No. 1-2, 1989, pp. 77-87.

801. Joshi, Pramila and Pande, P. C. "Ethnobotany of the Rajis of Kumaun Himalaya: a preliminary study". In Rishi-II: Utttaranchal Himalaya edited by M. P. Joshi, Shree Almora Book Depot, Almora, 1995, pp. 241-263.

802. Joshi, T. A. "Family planning through indigenous drugs and herbs". *Nagarjun,* Vol. 20, No. 2, 1976, pp. 17-20.

803. Joshi, Tankesh and Joshi, Muktesh "Ethno-ophiology-A traditional knowledge among the non- tribes of Bastar, Chhattisgarh". *Indian Journal of Traditional Knowledge,* Vol. 9, No. 1, 2010, pp. 137-139.

804. Joshi, Varun, Rawat, M. S. and Sharma, A. K. "Traditional knowledge of natural disaster mitigation and ethno medicine practices in Himalaya with special reference". *Indian Journal of Traditional Knowledge,* Vol. 10, No. 1, 2011, pp. 196-206.

805. Joyce, Christopher "Earthly goods: medicine-Hunting in the rainforest". New York, Little Brown and Co., 1994.

806. Juyal, S. P. and Uniyal, M. R. "Medicinal plants of Bhagirathi valley". *Nagarjun,* Vol. 10, No. 26, 1966.

807. Juyal, S. P. and Uniyal, M. R. "Medicinal plants of commercial and traditional importance in Bhilangana valley of Tehri Garhwal". *Nagarjun,* Vol. 10, 1960, pp. 26-36.

808. Kabiraj, S. "Fertility cult and trees". *Folklore,* 1965, pp. 162-169.

809. Kachare, S. V. and Suryawanshi, S. R. "Traditional medicines for diabetes from villages in Marathwada". *Ethnobotany,* Vol. 22, No. 1-2, 2010, pp. 149-151.

810. Kadel, Chitralekha and Jain, Ashok K. "Plants used in Ethnoveterinary Practices in Jhabua district, Madhya Pradesh". *Ethnobotany,* Vol. 18, No. 1-2, 2006, pp. 149-152.

811. Kagyung, R., Gajurel, P. R. and Rethy, P. "Ethnomedicinal plants used for gastro-intestinal diseases by Adi tribes of Dehang-Debang biosphere reserve in Arunachal Pradesh".

Indian Journal of Traditional Knowledge, Vol. 9, No. 3, 2009, pp. 496-501.

812. Kakar, D. N. "Anthropological research in medicine: an appraisal". Seminar on perspectives in Anthropological researches in India: planning for thc future researches and methodologies, New Delhi, Department of Anhtropology, Delhi Delhi University, 27 September -1 October 1985.

813. Kakar, D.N. "Folk and Modern medicine". New Delhi, New Asia Publishers, 1977.

814. Kakar, D.N. "Primary health care and traditional medical practitioners". New Delhi, Sterling,1985, p. 195

815. Kakar, D.N. "Primitive folk and modern medicine: a selected bibliography with special reference to community nutrition". Punjab Nutrition Development Project, Govt. of Punjab-CARE, 1973, p. 263.

816. Kakar, Sudhir "Shamans, Mystics and Doctors: A Psychological Inquiry into India and its Healing Traditions". New York, Alfred A. Knopf, 1982.

817. Kakati, L. N. and Doulo, V. "Indigenous knowledge system of zootherapeutic use by chakhesang tribe of Nagaland, India". *Journal of Human Ecology*, Vol. 13, No. 6, 2002, pp. 419-423.

818. Kakati, L. N., Ao, Bendang and Doulo, V. "Indigenous knowledge of zootherapeutic use of vertebrate origin by the Ao tribe of Nagaland". *Journal of Human Ecology*, Vol. 19, Vol. 3, 2006, pp. 163-167.

819. Kala, Chandra Prakash "Ethnomedicinal botany of the Apatani in the eastern Himalayan region of India". *Journal of Ethnobiology and Ethnomedicine*, Vol. 1, No. 11, 2005.

820. Kala, Chandra Prakash "Preserving ayurvedic herbal formulations by vaidyas: The traditional healers of the Uttaranchal Himalaya Region in India". *Herbal Gram,* No. 70, 2006, pp. 42-50.

821. Kala, Chandra Prakash and Rawat, G. S. "Human use and conservation status of wild medicinal herbs in the Bhyundar Valley, Western Himalaya". In Plant Diversity of the Himalaya edited by P. C. Pande and S. S. Samant, Gyanodaya Prakasan, Nainital, 2001, pp. 547-559.

822. Kala, Chandra Prakash, Farooquee, Nehal A. and Dhar, Uppeandra "Prioritization of medicinal plants on the basis of available knowledge, existing practices and use value status in Uttaranchal, India". *Biodiversity and Conservation,* Vol. 13, No.2, 2004, pp. 453-469.

823. Kalakoti, B. S. and Pangety, Y. P. S. "Ethnomedicine of Bhotiya tribe of Kumaun Himalaya, UA". *Bulletin of Medico-ethno-Botanical Research,* Vol. 9, 1988, pp. 11-20.

824. Kalita, Bhagaban, Choudhury, M. and Ojha, S. N. "Indigenous technical knowledge on pond construction and maintenance, fish seed transportation, and fish health management". *Indian Journal of Traditional Knowledge,* Vol. 3, No. 2, 2004, pp. 192-197.

825. Kalita, Bhagaban, Dutta, A. and Bhagabati, S.K. "Indigenous technical knowledge for fish harvesting in Karbi- Anglong district of Assam". *Indian Journal of Traditional Knowledge,* Vol. 9, No.2, 2009, pp. 252-255.

826. Kalita, Bhagaban, Dutta, Amalesh and Choudhury, M. "Herbal fish toxicant used by fishers of Karbi-anglong district, Assam". *Indian Journal of Traditional Knowledge,* Vol. 6, No. 2, 2007, 334-336.

827. Kalita, Dilip and Bonoranjan, Phukan "Folk medicines used by the Moran of Brahmaputra valley, Tinsukia district, Assam, India". *Indian Journal of Natural Products and Resources,* Vol. 8, No. 1, 2009, pp. 73-76.

828. Kalita, Dilip and Bora, Rajib Lochan "Some flok medicines from Lakhimpur district, Assam". *Indian Journal of Traditional Knowledge,* Vol. 7, No. 3, 2008, pp. 414-416.

829. Kalita, Dilip and Deb, Bikash "Folk medicines for some diseases prevalent in Lakhimpur district of Brahmaputra valley, Assam". *Indian Journal of Natural Products and Resources,* Vol. 5, No. 4, 2006, pp. 319-322.

830. Kalita, Dilip and Deb, Bikash "Some folk medicines used by the Sonowal Kacharis tribe of the Brahmaputra valley, Assam". *Indian Journal of Natural Products and Resources,* Vol. 3, No. 4, 2004, pp. 240-246.

831. Kalita, Dilip, Dutta, Manashi and Islam, Nazim Forid "Few plants and animals based folk medicines from Dibrugarh

district, Assam". *Indian Journal of Traditional Knowledge,* Vol. 4, No. 1, 2005, pp. 81-85.

832. Kalla, A. K. and Joshi, P. C. (eds.) "Tribal Health and medicines". New Delhi, Concept Publishing, 2004, p. 447.

833. Kalpesh, Ishnava, Rao, V. Rama and Parabia, F. M. "Ethnobotany of Little Rann of Kachchh, Gujarat". *Ethnobotany,* Vol. 16, No. 1-2, 2004, pp. 40-43.

834. Kamat, S. D. "Studies on medicinal plants and drugs in Dhanvantari-Nighantu". Delhi, Chaukhamba Sanskrit Pratishthan, 2002, p. 858.

835. Kamble, S. Y. and Prandhan, S. G. "Ethnobotany of 'Korkus' in Maharashtra". *Bulletin of the Botanical Survey of India,* Vol. 22, 1980, pp. 201-202.

836. Kamble, S. Y., More, T. N. and Patil, S. R. "Plants used by the tribes of northwest Maharashtra for the treatment of gastrointestinal disorders". *Indian Journal of Traditional Knowledge,* Vol. 7, No. 2, 2008, pp. 321-325.

837. Kamble, S. Y., Patil, S. R. and Sawant, P. S. "Studies on plants used in traditional medicine by Bhilla tribe of Maharashtra". *Indian Journal of Traditional Knowledge,* Vol. 9, No. 3, 2010, pp. 591-598.

838. Kamick, C. R. and Pathak, N. N. "Studies on the folklore and tribal medicines of India (Part 1): Tribal -lore of Himalayas (Rajori-Poonch areas)". *Nagarjun,* Vol. 26, 1983, pp. 100-103.

839. Kannan, R., Kubendran, A., Rani, M. Pitchai "Thokkam tratment: a study on adherence to ethno medicine in Meenatchipatti village". *The Oriental Anthropologist,* Vol. 11, No. 2, 2011, pp. 367-372.

840. Kanwar, Promila and Yadav, Dinesh "Indigenous animal healthcare practices of Kangra district, Himachal Pradesh". *Indian Journal of Traditional Knowledge,* Vol. 4, No. 2, 2005, pp. 164-168.

841. Kanwar, S. S., Gupta, M. K. and Katoch, Chhaya "Traditional fermented foods of Lahual and Spiti area of Himachal Pradesh". *Indian Journal of Traditional Knowledge,* Vol. 6 No.1, 2007, pp. 42-45.

842. Kapoor, S. L. and Mitra, R. "Herbal Durgs in Indian pharmaceutical industry". Lucknow, National Botanical Research Institute. 1979.

843. Kapur, S. K. "Traditionally important medicinal plants of Bhaderwah hills (Jammu Province) Part-II". In Ethnobotany and medicinal plants of Indian Sub-continent, edited by J.K. Maheshwari, Jodhpur, India Scientific Publishers, 2000.

844. Kapur, S.K. "Traditionally important medicinal plants of Bhaderwah hills Jammu Province III". In Ethnobotany and medicinal plants of Indian Sub-continent, edited by J.K. Maheshwari, Jodhpur, India Scientific Publishers, 2000.

845. Kapur, S. K. "Traditionally important medicinal plants of Bhaderwah hills Jammu Province-IV". In Ethnobotany and medicinal plants of Indian Sub-continent, edited by J.K. Maheshwari, Jodhpur, India Scientific Publishers, 2000.

846. Kapur, S. K. and Paviter Singh "Traditionally important medicinal plants of Udhampur district (Jammu Province) Part-I". In Ethnobotany and Medicinal plants of Indian Sub-continent, edited by J. K. Maheshwari, Jodhpur, India Scientific Publishers, 2000.

847. Kapur, S. K. and Sarin, Y. K. "Useful medicinal ferns of Jammu & Kashmir". *Indian Drugs*, Vol. 14, No. 7, 1977, p.136.

848. Kapur, S. K. and Srivastava, T. N. "Traditionally important medicinal plants of Udhampur district (Jammu Province) Part-II". In Ethnobotany and medicinal plants of Indian Sub-continent, edited by J. K. Maheshwari, Jodhpur, India Scientific Publishers, 2000.

849. Kar, Ajit, Choudhary, B. K. and Bandyopadhyay, N. G. "Evaluation of a few Indian Folk-medicinal Plants less known for their hypoglycaemic activity". *Ethnobotany*, Vol. 11, No. 1-2, 1999, pp. 18-21.

850. Kar, R. K. "Ethnomedicine and ribal health: An illustrative appraisal". In Tribal health and medicines, edited by A. K. Kalla and P. C. Joshi, New Delhi: Concept Publishing Co., 2004, pp. 376-390.

851. Kar, R. K. "Health Behavior among the Tribes of North-

East India: A Profile". *Journal of Indian Anthropology* Vol. 28, 1993, pp. 157-164.

852. Kar, Sujata, Mozumdar, Arupendra and Roy, Subrata K. "Age old health care system of rural Bengalese and meiteis of Cachar district in Assam: Beliefs and practices". *Man in India*, Vol. 89, No. 1-2, 2009, pp. 159-172.

853. Karlsson, B. G. "Anthropology and the Indigenous Slot: Claims to and Debates about Indigenous Peoples' Status in India". *Critique of Anthropology*, Vol. 23, No. 4, 2003, pp. 403-423.

854. Karna, M. N. "Etiology of disease: a sociological study in the rural context". *Man in India,* Vol. 56, pp. 50-56.

855. Karnick, C. R. "Studies on the drug plants used in Indian systems of medicine-"Akshadru" Melia azedarach". *Nagarjun*, Vol. 19, No. 4, 1975, pp. 36-37.

856. Karnick, C. R. "Studies on the drug plants used in Indian systems of medicine Khajur (Phoenix dactylifera L.)". *Nagarjun*, Vol. 20, No. 2, 1986, pp. 23.

857. Karnick, C. R. and Pathak, N. N. "Newer observations on folk-lore medicinal plants of Shiv-Khori forest area of the Western Himalayas". *Nagarjun*, Vol. 25, No. 7, 1982, pp. 156-162.

858. Karnick, C. R., Tiwari, K. C., Majumdar, R. and Bhattacharjee, S. "Newer ethno-botanical and folk-lore studies of some medicinal plants of Gauhati and surrounding areas". *Nagarjun*, Vol. 24, No. 1, 1981, pp. 240-245.

859. Karnik, S. R., Tathed, P. S. and Antarkar, D. S. "Antimalarial activity and clinical safety of traditionally used nyctanthes arbor - tristis linn". *Indian Journal of Traditional Knowledge,* Vol. 7, No. 2, 2008, pp. 330-334.

860. Karthickeyan, S. M. K. and Gajendran, K. "Indigenous technical know-how in the healthcare of domestic animals". *Indian Journal of Traditional Knowledge,* Vol. 4 No. 4, 2005, pp.462-463.

861. Katewa S. S. "Indigenous People and Forests: Perspectives of an Ethnobotanical study from Rajasthan (India)-Herbal Drugs: Ethnomedicine to modern medicine". Springer Berlin, 2009, pp. 33-56.

862. Katewa S. S., Chaudhary B. L. & Jain, A. "Folk herbal medicines from tribal area of Rajasthan, India". *Journal of Ethnopharmacology*, Vol. 92, No. 1, 2004, pp. 41-46.

863. Katewa, S. S. and Arora, Asha "Some plants in folk medicine of Udaipur district, Rajasthan". *Ethnobotany*, Vol. 9, No. 1-2, 1997, pp. 48-51.

864. Katewa, S.S. and Galav, P.K. "Additions to the traditional folk herbal medicines from Shekhawati region of Rajasthan". *Indian Journal of Traditional Knowledge,* Vol. 5, No. 4, 2006, pp. 491-500.

865. Katewa, S. S. and Galav, P. K. "Traditional herbal medicines from Shekhawati region of Rajasthan". *Indian Journal of Traditional Knowledge,* Vol. 4, No. 3, 2005, pp. 237-245.

866. Katewa, S. S., Chaudhary, B. L. and Jain, Anita "Traditional uses of plant biodiversity from aravalli hills of Rajasthan". *Indian Journal of Traditional Knowledge,* Vol. 2, No. 1, 2003, pp. 27-39.

867. Katewa, S. S., Choudhary, B. L. and Jain, Anita "Some plants in folk medicine of Rajsamand district (Rajasthan)". *Ethnobotany*, Vol. 13, 1-2, 2001, pp. 129-134.

868. Kattan, R. "A study in magic and medicine". *Vanyajati*, Vol. 3, No. 3, 1955, pp. 67-72.

869. Kaul M. K. "Medicinal plants of Kashmir and Ladakh, temperate and cold arid Himalaya". Indus Publishing Co., New Delhi, 1997, p. 123.

870. Kaul, M. K. "High altitude botanicals in integrative medicine- case studies from northwest Himalaya". *Indian Journal of Traditional Knowledge,* Vol. 9, No. 1, 2010, pp. 18-25.

871. Kaul, M. K. and Handa, S. S. "Medicinal plants on crossroads of Western Himalaya". In Himalayan medicinal Plants: Potential and Prospects, edited by S. S. Samant, U. Dhar and L. M. S. Palni, Gyanodaya Prakasan, Nainital, 2001, pp. 73-87.

872. Kaul, M. K., Singh V., Sharma, P. K. "Home remedies for arthritis in Kashmir Himalaya". *Arogya: Journal of Health Science*, Vol. 16, No. 81, 1990.

873. Kaushal, Sonia "Healing practices amongst the Gaddi tribe of Himachal Pradesh". In Tribal health and medicines, edited by A. K. Kalla and P. C. Joshi, New Delhi: Concept Publishing Co., 2004, pp. 301-310.

874. Kaushik, P. and Dhiman, A. K. "Some vadic medicinal plants". *Advances in Plant Science*, Vol. 9, No. 2, 1997, Supp. pp. 1-12.

875. Kaushik, Purushottam "Indigenous medicinal plants: including microbes and fungi". New Delhi, Today and Tomorrow's Printers, 1988, p. 243.

876. Keswani, N. H. "Science of medicine and physiological concepts in ancient and medieval India". New Delhi, S. K. Manchanda, 1974, p. 184.

877. Khan, C. G. and Mohd. Arif Ali "Relevance of ethnomedicine". *Man and Life,* Vol. 18, 1992, pp. 11-20.

878. Khan, J. B. and Singh, G. P. "Ethno- medicinal diversity of Churu district traditionally by rural people". Indian Journal of Fundamental and Applied Life Sciences, Vol. 2, No. 1, 2012, pp. 109-114. (http://www.cibtech.org/jls.htm)

879. Khan, M. S., Ahmad, Y. J., Satyanaryan, N. and Chagrai, S. A. "Botanical indentification of "Bhauphali', an important drug of the indigenous system of medicine". Journal of Research in Indian Medicine, Yoga and Homeopathy, Vol. 13, No.4, 1978, pp. 104-106.

880. Khan, P. M. "The Baids of Andhra Pradesh". Man of India, Vol. 46, 1966, pp. 14-32.

881. Khan, S. S. and Chaghatai, S. A., "Euphorbias of Bhopal and their medicinal utility". Chikitsa, Vol. 1, 1979, pp. 75-76.

882. Khan, S. S., Chaghtai, S. A. and Oommachan, M. "Ethnobotanical studies of certain rare medicinal plants of Bhopal". Journal of Science Research, Vol. 4, 1982, pp. 185-187.

883. Khan, S. S., Chaghtai, S. A. and Oommachan, M. "Medicinal plants of Rubiaceae of Bhopal- An ethnobotanical study". Journal of Science Research, Vol. 6, 1984, pp. 37-39.

884. Khan, S. S., Chaghtai, S. A., Siddiqui, M. S., Khan, S. M. & Iqbal, S. A. "Medicinal plants of central India". In ISMAP

International Conference, New Delhi (Abstract), 1989, p. 77.

885. Khan, S. S., Oomachan, M & Chaghtai, S. A. "Ethnobotany and ecology of certain medicinal plants of Bhopal". Proceedings of 69th Indian Science Congress, Part III (Abstract), 1982, p. 129.

886. Khan, Viquar A. and Khan, Athar A. "Herbal folklores for male sexual disorders and debilities in western Uttar Pradesh". *Indian Journal of Traditional Knowledge,* Vol. 4, No. 3, 2005, pp. 317-324.

887. Khan, Z. S., Khuroo, A.A. and Dar, G.H. "Ethnomedicinal survey of uri, Kashmir Himalaya". Indian Journal of Traditional Knowledge Vol. 3, No. 4, 2004, pp. 351-357.

888. Khandelwal, Sitaram "Ethnomedicine of Bhils in Rajasthan: Plants used in diarrhoea". Vanyajati, Vol. 46, No. 3, 1998, pp. 17-23.

889. Khanna, K. K. "Unreported Ethnomedicinal Uses of Plants from the Tribal and Rural Folklores of Gonda district, Uttar Pradesh". *Ethnobotany,* Vol. 14, No. 1-2, 2002, pp. 52-56.

890. Khanna, K. K. and Kumar, Ramesh "Ethnomedicinal Plants used by the Gujjar Tribe of Saharanpur district, Uttar Pradesh". *Ethnobotany,* Vol. 12, No. 3, 2000, pp. 17-22.

891. Khanna, K. K., Dongarwar, N. M. and Makde, K. H. "Unreported Ethnomedicinal Uses of Canscora Decussata (Gentianaceae) among the Tribals of Maharashtra". *Ethnobotany,* Vol. 17, No. 1-2, 2005, pp. 187-188,

892. Khanna, K.K., Mudgal, V., Shukla, G. & Srivastava, P. K. "Unreported ethnomedicinal uses of plants from Mirzapur district, Uttar Pradesh" In Ethnobotany and medicinal plants of Indian Sub-continent, edited by J. K. Maheshwari, Jodhpur, India Scientific Publishers, 2000.

893. Khanna, K. K., Shukla, G. and Mudgal, V. "New traditional medicinal uses of plants from Jalaun district, Uttar Pradesh". In Ethnobotany and medicinal plants of Indian Sub-continent, edited by J. K. Maheshwari, Jodhpur, India Scientific Publishers, 2000.

894. Khanna, K. K., Srivastava, P. K. & Mudgal, V. "Noteworthy medicinal plant uses from rural folklore of Raebareli district,

Uttar Pradesh". In Ethnobotany and medicinal plants of Indian Sub-continent, edited by J. K. Maheshwari, Jodhpur, India Scientific Publishers, 2000.

895. Khanna, K. K., Srivastava, P. K., Shukla, G. & Mudgal, V. "Unknown traditional uses of plants as veterinary medicines from Uttar Pradesh". Proceedings of the National Academy of Sciences of India 63B, IV, 1993.

896. Khare, R. S. "Dava, Daktar and Dua: Anthropology of practiced medicine in India". Social Science and Medicine, Vol. 43, No. 5, 1996, pp. 837-848.

897. Khare, R. S. "Folk medicine in a north Indian village: Some further motos and obervations", In Main currents Indian sociology, Vol. 4, edited by Giriraj Gupta New Delhi, Vikas Publishing, 1981, pp. 125-147.

898. Khare, R. S. "Folk medicine in a North Indian Village". Human Organisation, Vol. 22, 1963, pp. 36-40.

899. Kharkongor, P. and Joseph, J. "Folk lore medico-botany of rural Khasi and Jaintia tribes in Meghalaya". In Glimpses of Indian Ethnobotany, edited by S. K. Jain, New Delhi, Oxford and IBH, 1980, pp. 124-136.

900. Khatoon, Sayyada and Goel, Anil K.A brief review on ethno-medicines used in cognitive and brain disorders". *Ethnobotany,* Vol. 22, No. 1-2, 2010, pp. 55-66.

901. Khatua, Nilanjan "Indigenous health practices among the Hill Korwa of Chhattisgarh". In Primitives tribes in contemporary India (in 2 Vols.) edited by Sarit K. Chaudhary and Suchita Sen Chaudhary, New Delhi, Mittal Publicatiosn, 2005.

902. Khetwal, K. S. and Verma, D. L. "Chemical screening of some potential medicinal plants of high altitude Kumaun Himalayan glaciers". Indian Drugs, Vol. 28, No, 2, 1990, pp. 99-100.

903. Khongsai, M., Saikia, S. P. and Kayang, H. "Ethnomedicinal plants used by different tribes of Arunachal Pradesh". *Indian Journal of Traditional Knowledge,* Vol. 10, No. 3, 2011, pp. 541-546.

904. Khory, Rustomjee Naserwanjee "Materia medica of India and their therapeutics". Delhi, Neeraj, 1985, p. 809.

905. Khory, Rustomjee Naserwanjee "Principles and Practice of Ayurvedic Medicine (in 2 Vols.)". Delhi, Biothech Books, 2004, p. 1056.

906. Khullar, S. P. "Ferns in medicine and how to identify them". In Himalayan medicinal plants: Potential and prospects edited by S. S. Samant, U. Dhar and L.M.S. Palni, Gyanodaya Prakashan, Nainital, 2001, pp. 65-73.

907. Khurana, I. "Best kept sacred". Down to Earth, Vol. 6, No. 23, 1998, pp. 34-35.

908. Kimothi, G. P and Shah, B. C. L. "Some medicinal plants of Gopeshwar-Tungnath region of Uttar Pradesh". Ancient Science Life, Vol. 8, 1989, pp. 283-292.

909. King, G. "Famine foods of Marwar". Proceedings of Asiatic Society Bengal, Vol. 38, 1869, pp. 116-122.

910. Kingston, C. and others "Indigenous knowledge of using medicinal plants in treating skin disease in Kanyakumari district, Southern India". *Indian Journal of Traditional Knowledge,* Vol. 8, No. 2, 2009, pp. 196-200.

911. Kingston, Jeremy "Healing without medicine". London, Aldus Books, 1976, p.144.

912. Kirtikar, K. R. "Folk-lore of Indian plants". Journal of Bombay Natural History Sociology, Vol. 3, 1886, pp. 54-63.

913. Kirtikar, K. R. and Basu, B. D. "Indian medicinal plants – with illustrations". 2nd edition, Oriental Enterprises, Dehradoon, 2001.

914. Kirtikar, K. R. and Basu, B. D. "Indian medicinal plants, (in 4 Vols.)". International Book Distributors, Dehradun, 1981.

915. Kiruba, S., Jeeva, S. and Das, S. Sam Manohar "Bomboo seeds as a means to sustenance of the indigenous community". *Indian Journal of Traditional Knowledge,* Vol. 6, No. 1, 2007, pp.199-203.

916. Kleinman, A. Eisebergi and Good, B. "Culture: illness and cure, clinically lessons from anthropologic and cross - cultural research". Annals of internal medicine, Vol. 88, 1978, pp. 251-258.

917. Kleinman, Arthur, and Kunstadter, Peter "Introduction". In Culture and Healing in Asian Societies: Anthropological,

Psychiatric and Public Health Studies edited by Arthur Kleinman, Peter Kunstadter, E. Russell Alexander, and James L. Gale, Boston, G. K. Hall & Co 1978, pp. 1-13.

918. Kloos, H. "Disease concepts and medicinal practices in relations to malaria among fever cases in Addis Abada". Ethnomedicine, Vol. 2, 1973, pp. 229-253.

919. Kobarfard, F., Velayati, A., Mosaddegh, M., Massjedi, M. R. and Farnia, P. "Tuberculosis and traditional medicine: fighting the oldest infectious disease, using the oldest source of medicine". Iranian Journal of Pharmaceutical Research, Vol. 3, Suppl. 2, 13, 2004.

920. Kochar, Vijay and others "Linking the folk health system to rural healty services". Swasth Hind, February, Vol. 23, No. 2, 1979, p.15.

921. Koppula, Hemadri "A treatise on tribal medicine". Koppula Hemadri, 2011, p. 228.

922. Kotecha, Vaidya Mita "Concept of Lekhana in ayurveda". Jaipur, Publication Scheme, 2000, p. 122.

923. Koul, Ashwani, Gangar, Subhash Chander, Sandhir, Vandana "Pitfalls in journey from traditional to modern medicine". Indian Journal of Natural Products and Resources, Vol. 4, No. 1, 2005, pp. 6-13.

924. Koul, S. C. "Some wild flowers of Kashmir and their indigenous use". Journal of Bombay Natural History Society, Vol. 42, 1941, pp. 452-454.

925. Krippner, S. "Models of Ethnomedicinal Healing". Paper Presented at the Ethnomedicine Conferences, Munich, Germany. April 26–27 and October 11–12, 2003.

926. Krippner, S. and Welch, P. "Spiritual dimension of healing: From tribal Shamanism to contemporary healthcare". New York, Irvington, 1992.

927. Krishnamurthy, K. H. "Onion and garlic". Delhi, Books for All, p. 112.

928. Krishnamurthy, K. H. "Wealth of Susruta". Coimbatore, International Institute of Ayurveda, 1991, p. 582.

929. Kshatriva, G. K. "Tribal health in India: Perspectives in medical anthropology". In Tribal health and medicines, edited by A. K. Kalla and P. C. Joshi, New Delhi, Concept Publishing Co., pp. 17-45.

930. Kshirsagar, R. D. and Singh, N. P. "Less-known Ethnomedicinal uses of plants reported by Jenu kuruba tribe of Mysore district, Southern India". *Ethnobotany,* Vol. 12, No. 1-2, 2000, pp. 118-122.

931. Kshirsagar, R. D. and Singh, N. P. "Less-known Ethnomedicinal uses of plants in Coorg district of Karnataka state, Southern India". *Ethnobotany,* Vol. 12, No. 1-2, 2000, pp. 12-16.

932. Kulharni, L.B., "The drugs of Sirsi and Kappat Hills". Journal of Bombay Natural History Society, Vol. 19, 1909, pp. 574-584.

933. Kulkarni, C.G. and Deshpande, Adwait "Folk therapies of Katkaris from Maharashtra". *Indian Journal of Traditional Knowledge,* Vol. 10, No. 3, 2011, pp. 554-558.

934. Kulkarni, D.K. and Kumbhojkar, M. S. "Kitchen Garden Plants of Mahadeokoli Tribe in Maharashtra". *Ethnobotany,* Vol. 5, No. 1-2, 1993, pp. 119-127.

935. Kulkarni, D.K., Agte, V. V. and Kumbhojkar, M. S. "Leafy vegetables consumed by Mahadeokoli tribe in Western Maharashtra with their nutritional potential". *Ethnobotany,* Vol. 15, No. 1-2, 2003, pp. 34-38.

936. Kulkarni, D. K., Kumbhojkar, M. S. and Upadhye, A. "Ethnobiological resources used in traditional medicines by Mahadeo Koli tribe from western Maharashtra". Flora and Fauna, Vol. 1, No. 1, 1995, pp. 65-66.

937. Kumar Vivek and Rao, R. R. "Some interesting indigenous beverages among the tribals of Central India". *Indian Journal of Traditional Knowledge,* Vol. 6, No. 1, 2007, pp. 141-143.

938. Kumar, Akhilesh, Tewari, D.D. and Tewari, J.P. "Ethnomedicinal knowledge among Tharu tribe of devipatan division". *Indian Journal of Traditional Knowledge,* Vol. 5, No. 3, 2006, pp. 310-313.

939. Kumar, Anand "Some ethnomedicinal plants of the Murias of the Indravati Tiger Reserve, Bastar, (Madhya Pradesh)". In Ethnobotany and medicinal plants of Indian Sub-continent, edited by J. K. Maheshwari, Jodhpur, India Scientific Publishers, 2000.

940. Kumar, Anil "Medicine and the raj: British medical policy

in India 1835-1911". Walnut Creek, CA: Alta Mira Press, 1998,

941. Kumar, Deepak "Health and medicine in British India and Dutch Indies: A comparative study". In Asian medicine and globalization, edited by Joseph S. Alter, Philadelphia, University of Pennsylvania Press, 2005, pp. 78-87.

942. Kumar, Deepak "Medical encounters in British India, 1820-1920". *Economic and Political Weekly,* Vol. 32, No. 4, 1997, pp. 166-170.

943. Kumar, Deepak "Unequal contenders, uneven ground: Medical encounters in British India, 1982-1920". In Western medicine as contested knowledge edited by Andrew Cunningham and Bridie Andrews, Manchester, Manchester University Press, 1997, pp. 172-190.

944. Kumar, J. K., Bhatnagar, S.P. and Gupta, R. N. "Fuzzy inference system: A marvelous tool in conservation of traditional knowledge". Pharma Times, Vol. 36, 2004, pp. 20-20.

945. Kumar, J. K., Bhatnagar, S. P. and Gupta, R. N. "Neural fuzzy systems: A link between evaluation traditional medicines and complementary medicine". Pharma Times, Vol. 37, 2005, pp. 18-24.

946. Kumar, K. Jayaram "Bottle Necks in Standardization of Traditional System of Medicines". Research Journal of Medicinal plants, Vol. 5, No. 4, 2011, pp. 443 - 447.

947. Kumar, Kaushal "Observation on some phytodiversity resources used as food and medicine by Santhal and Paharia community of Bihar". Vanyajati, Vol. 47, No. 4, 1999, pp. 21-22.

948. Kumar, Kaushal and Goel, A. K. "Frequently used ethno-medicinal plants of Bihar". *Journal of Economic and Taxonomic Botany,* Vol. 23, 1999, pp. 645-649.

949. Kumar, Kaushal and Goel, A.K. "Frequently used ethno-medicinal plants of Bihar". In Ethnobotany and medicinal plant of Indian subcontinent, edited by J.K. Maheshwari, Saujanya Books, Jodhpur, 2003, p. 672.

950. Kumar, Rajesh and Bharati, Avinash Kumar "Folk veterinary medicines in Jalaun district of Uttar Pradesh,

India". *Indian Journal of Traditional Knowledge,* Vol. 11, No. 2, 2012, pp. 288-295.

951. Kumar, S. and Chauhan, A. K. S. "Less-known medicinal uses of plant species in Keoladeo National Park, Bharatpur, Rajasthan". *Ethnobotany,* Vol. 18, No. 1-2, 2006, pp. 153-156.

952. Kumar, S. and Chauhan, A.K.S. "Medicinal plants used by local inhabitants in Bharatpur district, Rajasthan". *Ethnobotany,* Vol. 17, No. 1-2, 2005, pp. 179-183.

953. Kumar, Sanjay "Indigenous communities' knowledge of local ecological services". *Economic and Political Weekly,* Vol. 36, No. 30, 2001, pp. 2859-2869.

954. Kumar, Suresh, Goyal, Sangeeta and Parveen, Farzana "Ethno-medico-botany of household remedies of Kolayat tehsil in Bikaner district, Rajasthan". *Indian Journal of Traditional Knowledge,* Vol. 2, No. 4, 2003, pp. 357-365.

955. Kumar, Suresh, Goyal, Sangeeta and Parveen, Farzana "Ethnoveterinary plants in Indian arid zone". *Ethnobotany,* Vol. 16, No. 1-2, 2004, pp. 91-95.

956. Kumar, Suresh, Parveen, Farzana and Goyal, Sangeeta "Indigenous herbal coolants for combating heat stress in the hot Indian arid zone". *Indian Journal of Traditional Knowledge,* Vol. 7, No. 4, 2008, pp. 679-682.

957. Kumar, T. Dharma Chandra and Pullaiah, T. "Ethno-medicinal uses of some plants of Mahabubnagar district, Andhra Pradesh, India", In Ethnobotany and medicinal plant of Indian subcontinent, edited by J.K. Maheshwari, Saujanya Books, Jodhpur, 2003, p. 672.

958. Kumar, Vivek and Rao, R.R. "Some plant beverages used in traditional medicine". *Ethnobotany,* Vol. 13, No. 1-2, 2001, pp. 36-39.

959. Kumar, Viviek and Sikarwar, R. L. S. "Plants used as fish poison by tribals of Surguja district in Chhattisgarh, India". *Ethnobotany,* Vol. 15, No. 1-2, 2003, pp. 87-89.

960. Kumar, Y., Fancy, S. and Rao, R. R. "Further contribution to ethnobotancy of Meghalaya: Plants used by 'War Jaintia' of Jaintia hill district". *Journal of Economic Taxomonic Botany,* Vol. 11, 1987, pp. 65-70.

961. Kumar, Y., K. Haridasan and R. R. Rao, "Ethnobotanical notes on certain medicinal plants among some Garo people around Balphakrah Santuary in Meghalaya". *Bulletin of the Botanical Survey of India*, Vol. 22, 1980, pp. 161-165.

962. Kumaran, T. Vasantha, Jaganathan, R. and Anbazhahan, N. "Indigenous or local knowledge for sustainable bio-diversity and food security in the tribal Kolli Hills". *South Indian Folklorist*, Vol. 2, No. 1, 1998, pp. 7-26.

963. Kurian, J.C. and Bhanu, B.V. "Ethnomedicine: The nomadic vaidus of Maharashtra". *The Eastern Anthropologist*, Vol. 33, 1980, pp. 71-78.

964. Kurian, J.C. and Tribhuwan, Robin D. "Traditional medical practitioners of the Sahyadri". *The Eastern Anthropologist,* Vol. 43, No. 3, 1990, pp. 251-258.

965. Kuriyan, John "Traditional practioners of medicine in a tribal area: Their integration with the existing health care system". *Health and Population perspectives and issues,* Vol. 8, No. 2, 1985, pp. 103-107.

966. Kuriyan, John "Traditional practitioners of medicines in a tribal area: Their integration with the existing health care system" *Tribal Research Bulletin,* Vol. 9, No. 1, 1986, pp. 30-32.

967. Kurup, A.M. "Glimpses of life and culture of the tribes of Madhya Pradesh". *Vanyajati*, Vol. 10, No.4, 1962, pp. 134-145.

968. Kutumbiah, P. "Ancient Indian medicine". Bombay, Orient Longman, 1962, p. 233.

969. Lachungpa, Usha "Indigenous lifestyles and biodiversity conservation issues in North Sikkim". *Indian Journal of Traditional Knowledge,* Vol. 1, No. 1, 2009, pp. 51-55.

970. Lad, Vasant "Ayurveda the science of self-healing: a practical guide". Delhi, Motilal Banarasidass, 1984, p.175.

971. Lakra, Valeria, Singh, M.K. and Sinha, Rekha "Indigenous technology of tribal farmers in Jharkhand". *Indian Journal of Traditional Knowledge,* Vol. 9, No. 2, 2010, pp. 261-263.

972. Lakshamanan, K.K. and Sankaranarayanan, A.S. "Some folklore medicines in the remote hemlets, Dhoomanoor and Champukrari of Anai Katty hills, Coimbatore, Tamil

Nadu". *Indian Journal of Forestry*, Vol. 11, 1988, pp. 217-219.

973. Lal, B. H. Dasmana and Nigam, R. K. "A contribution to the medicinal plants lore of Garhwal region". *Himalayan Research and Development,* Vol. 8, No. 182, 1989, pp. 24-30.

974. Lal, Brij and Dube, V.P. "A survey of plant ethnomedicine of Amarkantak plateau in central India". *Agricultural and Biological Research*, Vol. 8, No. 1, 1992, pp. 29-37.

975. Lal, Brij and Singh, K. N. "Indigenous herbal remedies used to cure skin disorders by the natives of Lahaul - Spiti in Himachal pradesh". *Indian Journal of Traditional Knowledge,* Vol. 7, No. 2, 2008, pp. 237-241.

976. Lal, Brij and Upreti, D. K. "Ethnobotanical notes on three Indian lichens". *Lachenologist*, Vol. 27, No. 1, 1995, pp. 77-79.

977. Lal, Brij, "Traditional remedies for bone fracture among the tribals of M. P. India". *Bulletin of the tribal Research and Development Institute*, Vol. 15, No. 1-2, 1987.

978. Lal, Chaman and Verma, L. R. "Indigenous technological knowledge on soil and water management from Himachal Himalaya". *Indian Journal of Traditional Knowledge,* Vol. 7, No. 3, 2008, pp. 485-493.

979. Lal, Chaman and Verma, L. R. "Use of certain bio-products for insect-pest control". *Indian Journal of Traditional Knowledge,* Vol. 5, No. 1, 2006, pp. 79-82.

980. Lal, S.D. "Change in the dietary of habits of physique of aboriginals in santal parganas district, Bihar". *Journal of Indian Medical Research,* 1957, pp. 167-179.

981. Lal, S. D. and Lata, K. "Plants used by the Bhat community for regulating fertility". *Economic Botany*, Vol. 34, 1980, pp. 273-275.

982. Lal, S.D. and Yadav, B. K. "Folk medicine of Kurukshetra District Haryana". *Economic Botany,* Vol. 37, 1983, pp. 299-305.

983. Lal, V.K. and Tewari, V.P. "Sitajatu ka vaigyoik vivechan". *Sachitra Ayurveda*, May 1977. [Hind]

984. Lalfakzuala, R., Lalrammghinglova, H. and Kayang, H.

"Ethnobotanical usages of plants in western Mizoram *Indian Journal of Traditional Knowledge,* Vol. 6, No. 3, 2007, pp. 486-493.

985. Laloo, R.C., Kharlukhi, L. and Jeeva, S. "Status of medicinal plants in the disturbed and the undisturbed sacred forests of Meghalaya, northeast India: Population structure and regeneration efficacy of some important species". *Current Science*, Vol. 90, No. 2, 2006, pp. 225-232.

986. Lalramnghinglova, H. "Ethnobotanical study on the edible plants of Mizoram". *Ethnobotany,* Vol. 14, No. 1-2, 2002, pp. 23-33.

987. Lalramnghinglova, H. "Plants used in ethnoveterinary medicine including treatment of snake and insect bites in Mizoram". *Ethnobotany,* Vol. 23, No. 1-2, 2011, pp. 57-63.

988. Lalramnghinglova, J. H. "Ethnobotany of Mizoram—a preliminary survey". In Ethnobotany and medicinal plants of Indian Sub-continent, edited by J.K. Maheshwari, Jodhpur, India Scientific Publishers, 2000.

989. Lalramnghinglova, J. H. and Jha, L.K. "Ethnomedicine from Mizoram: North East India". *Ethnobotany,* Vol. 9, No. 1-2, 1997, pp. 105-111.

990. Lamba, Rajni and Mehta, Shalina "Priorities in Indian medicine: A tribal perspective". Indian Anthropologist, Vol. 25, No. 2, 1995, pp. 1-12.

991. Lambert J., Shrivastava, J. and Vietmeyer, N. "Medicinal plants, rescuing a global heritage". The World Bank, Washington DC, 1997, p. 61.

992. Lambert, Helen "Plural Traditions?: Folk Therapeutics and "English" medicine in Rajasthan". In Western medicine as contested knowledge edited by Andrew Cunningham and Bridie Andrews, Manchester: Manchester University Press. 1997, pp. 191-211.

993. Lambert, Helen "The cultural logic Indian medicine: Prognosis and etiology in Rajasthani popular therapeutics". Social Science and Medicine, Vol. 34, No. 10, 1992, pp. 1069-1076.

994. Landy J. (ed.) "Culture disease and healing: studies in medical anthropology". London, Collier Macmillan Publishers, 1977.

995. Langford, Jean M. "Traces of folk medicine in Jaunpur". *Cultural Anthropology*, Vol. 18, No. 3, 2003, pp. 271-303.

996. Lanusunep and Jamir, N. S. "Folk-medicinal herbs used by the Sumi- Naga tribes of Zunheboto district, Nagaland". *Pleione,* Vol. 4, No. 2, 2010, pp. 215-220.

997. Lashari, Mohammad Saleh "Traditional and modern medicine- is a marriage possible". *World Health Forum,* Vol. 5, 1984.

998. Leavitt, John "Oracular therapy in the Kumaon Hills: A question of rationality". *Indian Anthropologist*, Vol. 16, No. 1, 1986, pp. 71-79.

999. Leiban, R.W. "Medical anthropology". In the Handbook of Social and cultural anthropology edited by J. I. Honigmann Rand Menally and Company, 1973.

1000. Lekshmi, P.S. Swathi, and Dinesh Babu, A. P. "Indigenous technical knowledge and ancient proverbs of the coastal fisher folk of Kerala and their implications". *Indian Journal of Traditional Knowledge,* Vol. 8, No. 2, 2009, pp. 296-297.

1001. Lemley, Brad "Alternative medicine man: why so many doctors hate Andrew Weil". Discover, Vol. 20, No. 8, 1999, pp. 56-63.

1002. Leslie, C. "Modern India's ancient medicine". Transaction, Vol. 68, 1967, pp. 46-55.

1003. Lodha, R. and Bagga, A. "Traditional Indian systems of medicine". *Annals of the Academy of Medicine, Singapore,* Vol. 29, No. 1, 2000, pp. 37-41.

1004. Loudon, J.B. "Social anthropology and medicine (ASA monograph -13)". London, Academic Press, 1976.

1005. Lovelock, James "Healing Gaia: practical medicine for the planet". New York, Harmony Books, 1991, p. 192.

1006. Luxae E. "800 year old book of Indian medicine and formulas", London, 1937.

1007. M. Cyrilnayagam, R. Ravi & R. Kandasamy "Plants used by Kattunayakkas for stupefying fishes". In Ethnobotany and medicinal plants of Indian sub-continent, edited by J.K. Maheshwari, Jodhpur, India Scientific Publishers, 2000.

1008. Madan, T.N. "Doctor and Society", New Delhi, Vices Publishing House, 1980.

1009. Madan, T.N. "Who chose modern medicine and why". *Economic and Political Weekly,* Vol. 37, 1969, pp. 1475-1484.

1010. Mahajan, S.K. "Traditional herbal remedies among the tribes of Bijagarh of West Nimar district, Madhya Pradesh". *Indian Journal of Traditional Knowledge,* Vol. 6, No. 2, 2007, pp. 375-377.

1011. Mahanta, K. C. "A study of ethno-medicines in Assam: A general perspective". *Journal of Human Ecology*, Vol. 6, No. 2, 1995, pp. 105-117.

1012. Mahapatra, A.K. and Panda, P.K. "Ethno-pharmacological knowledge of Juang and Munda tribes of Eastern India". *International Journal of Sustainable Development and World Ecology,* Vol. 9, No. 2, 2002, 151-158.

1013. Mahapatra, L. K. "Concept of health among the tribal population groups of India and its socio- economic and socio-cultural correlates". In Tribal health in India edited by Salil Basu, Delhi, Manak Publications, 1994, pp. 1-12.

1014. Mahapatra, Sitakant, "Modernization and ritual: identity and chane in santal society". Calcutta, Oxford University Press, 1986.

1015. Mahato, Ashwini Kumar and Mahato, Pushpa "Ethnobotanical wealth of Chhotanagpur plateau- IV. Some medicinal plants used against intestinal worms". In Ethnobotany and medicinal plants of Indian Sub-continent, edited by J.K. Maheshwari, Jodhpur, India Scientific Publishers, 2000.

1016. Mahawar, Madan Mohan and Jaroli, D.P. "Animals and their products utilized as medicines by the inhabitants surrounding the Ranthambore National Park, India". *Journal of Ethnobiology and Ethno-medicine*, Vol. 2, No. 46, 2006.

1017. Mahawar, Madan Mohan and Jaroli, D. P. "Traditional knowledge on zootherapeutic uses by the Saharia tribe of Rajasthan, India". *Journal of Ethnobiology and Ethno-medicine,* Vol. 3, No. 25, 2007.

1018. Mahawar, Nilanjan "Nomadic medicine men: The Mitta Gonds of central India". *The India Magazine*, Vol. 6, No. 7, 1986, pp. 28-33.

1019. Mahdihassan, M. "Treatment of the system as whole as recognised in traditional medicines and its psychogenesis". *SHM* Vol. 8, No. 3&4, 1984, pp. 107-114.

1020. Maheshwari, J. K and Singh, J. P., "Plants used in ethnomedicine by the Kols of Allahabad district, Uttar Pradesh", *Bulletin of Medico-Ethn-obotanic Research*, Vol. 5, 1984, pp. 105-121.

1021. Maheshwari, J.K. (ed.) "Ethnobotany and medicinal plants of Indian sub-continent". Jodhpur, India Scientific Publishers, 2000, p. 672.

1022. Maheshwari, J.K. "Ethnobotanical documentation of primitive tribes of Madhya Pradesh, India". In Ethnobotany and medicinal plants of Indian Sub-continent, edited by J.K. Maheshwari, Jodhpur, India Scientific Publishers, 2000.

1023. Maheshwari, J.K. and Dwivedi, R.P. "Ethnomedicinal plants of Bharia tribe of Patalkot Valley, Chindwara District, M.P.". In Indigenous medicinal plants: including microbes and fungi edited by Purshotam Kaushik, Today and tomorrow's printers and Publishers, New Delhi, 1988, pp. 139-156.

1024. Maheshwari, J.K. and others (eds.) "Ethnobotany in India". Jodhpur, Scientific, 1993, p. 499.

1025. Maheshwari, J.K. and Singh, J.P. "Contribution to the ethnobotany of Bhoxa tribe of Bijnor and Pauri Garhwal districts, U. P.". *Journal of Economic Taxonomic Botany,* Vol. 5, 1984, pp. 251-259.

1026. Maheshwari, J.K. and Singh, J.P. "Plants used in magico-religious beliefs by the Kols of Uttar Pradesh: A study". *Folklore*, Vol. 26, No. 9, 1985, pp. 170-173.

1027. Maheshwari, J.K., Kalakoti, B.S. and Brijlal "Ethnomedicine of Bhil tribe of Jhabua district, M.P.". *Ancient Science of Life,* Vol. 5, No. 4, 1986, pp. 255-261.

1028. Maheshwari, J.K., Sikarwar, R.L.S. and Painuli, R.M. "Plants used in tribal medicine in the Dangs District of Gujarat". *Aryavaidyan*, Vol. 7, No. 4, 1994, pp. 201-205.

1029. Maheshwari, J.K., Singh, K.K. and Saha, S. "Ethnomedicinal uses of plants by Tharus Kheri district,

Uttar Pradesh". *Bulletin of Medico-Ethno-botanic Research,* Vol. 1, 1980, pp. 318-337.

1030. Maheshwari, J. K., Singh, K. K. and Saha, S. "The Ethnobotany of Tharus of Kheri district, Uttar Pradesh". Lucknow, National Botanical Research Institute, 1981.

1031. Maheswari, J. K. and Singh, Harish "Herbal remedies of Bhoxas of Nainital district, UP". *Aryavaidyan*, Vol. 4, No. 1, 1990.

1032. Mahindru, S.N. "Spices in Indian life (6500 B.C.-1950 A.D.): a comprehensive and critical narration about the role of spices in Indian life". New Delhi, Sultan Chand and Sons, 1982, p. 215.

1033. Maikhuri, R.K., Nautiyal, Suneel & Rao, K. S. "Nanda Devi jaiv mandal aarkshit chetra (Biosphere Reserve) mai auoshdhi padpo ke paramparagat krishi taknik ". GBPIHED, Koshi-Katarmal, Almora, 1991. [Hindi]

1034. Mairh, Ashutosh kumar, Mishra, P.K. and Kumar, Jyoti "Traditional botanical wisdom of Birhore tribes of Jharkhand". *Indian Journal of Traditional Knowledge,* Vol. 9, No. 3, 2009, pp. 467-470.

1035. Maiti, A. and Manna, C. K. "Some ethnomedicines used by the Santal of Baghmundi: Ajodhya hill region of Puruliya district, West Bengal". *Ethnobotany,* Vol. 12, No. 1-2, 2000, pp. 72-76.

1036. Maiti, D.C., Chauhan, A. S., Maiti, G. "Ethnonotanical notes on some unexploited plants used by Lepchas and Nepalese Communities of North Sikkim". In Ethnobotany and medicinal plants of India and Nepal, Vol. 1, edited by V. Singh, A.P. Jain, Jodhpur, India, Scientific Publishers, 2003, pp. 325-332.

1037. Maiti, S. and Mishra, T. K. "Anti-venom drugs of Santals, Savars and Mahatos of Midnapore district of West Bengal, India". *Ethnobotany,* Vol. 12, No. 1-2, 2000, pp. 77-80.

1038. Maity, D., Pradhan, N. and Chauhan, A.S. "Folk uses of some medicinal plants from North Sikkim". *Indian Journal of Traditional Knowledge,* Vol. 3, No. 1, 2004, pp. 66-71.

1039. Majhi, Jagannath and Sharma, B. V. "Ethnomedical practitioners and their clients among the Kondhs". *Man in India,* Vol. 84, 1-2, 2004, pp. 99-107.

1040. Majhi, Sullip Kumar "Indigenous technical knowledge for control of insect pest and livestrok disorders". *Indian Journal of Traditional Knowledge,* Vol. 7, No. 3, 2008, pp. 463-465.

1041. Majumdar, D. N. "Affairs of a tribe: A study in tribal dynamics". Lucknow, Universal publishers, 1950.

1042. Majumdar, D.N. "An account of magico-religious rites and beliefs of the Rongdani Rabha". Bulletin of the Anthropological Survey of India, Vol. 17, No. 3, 1968, pp. 245-256.

1043. Majumdar, D.N. "Races and cultures of India". Bombay, Asia Publishing House, 1961.

1044. Majumdar, G.P. "Vanaspati-plant and plant life as in Indian-treatises of traditions". Calcutta, 1927.

1045. Majumdar, Koushik and Datta, B. K. "Leucas biflora (Vahl) R. Br.(Lamiaceae): A new distributional record and its less known ethno-medicinal usage from Tripura". *Indian Journal of Traditional Knowledge,* Vol. 10, No. 3, 2011, pp. 575-577.

1046. Majumdar, Koushik, Saha, Reema and Datta, B.K. "Medicinal plants prescribed by different tribal and non-tribal medicine men of Tripura state". *Indian Journal of Traditional Knowledge,* Vol. 5, No. 4, 2006, pp. 559-562.

1047. Majumder, R. K., Tiwari, C., Bhattacharjee, S. and Nair, A.R. "Some folklore medicine from Assam and Meghalaya". *Pharmaceutical Biology*, Vol. 16, No. 4, 1978, pp. 185-189.

1048. Malhotra, C. L. and Balodi, B. "Medicinal plants of Alpine region of Gori valley, Kumaon", *Journal of Science Research Plant Medicine*, Vol. 5, 1984, pp.1-8.

1049. Malhotra, C.L. and Balodi, B. "Wild medicinal plants in the use of Johari tribals". *Journal of Economic and Taxonomic Botany,* Vol. 5, No. 4, 1984, pp. 881-883.

1050. Malhotra, C.L. and Bashu, D. "A preliminary survey of plants resources of medicinal and aromatic value from Almora". *Journal of Economic and Taxonomic Botany*, Vol. 5, 1984, pp. 859-864.

1051. Malhotra, S.K. and Mitra, S. "Some useful and medicinal plants of Chandrapur district (Maharashtra state)". *Bulletin of the botanical Survey of India*, Vol. 15, 1973, pp. 13-21.

1052. Malik, Akhtar H., Khuroo, Anzar A. and Dar, G. H. "Ethno-medicinal uses of some plants in the Kashmir Himalaya". *Indian Journal of Traditional Knowledge,* Vol. 10, No. 2, 2011, pp. 362-366.

1053. Maliya, S.D. "Some new or less-known folk medicines of district Bahraich, Uttar Pradesh, India-II". *Ethnobotany,* Vol. 16, No. 1-2, 2004, pp. 113-115.

1054. Maliya, S.D. "Use of some Indian plants in folk medicines of Nepal". *Ethnobotany,* Vol. 17, No. 1-2, 2005, pp. 202-204.

1055. Maliya, S.D. and Singh, K.K. "Some new or less-known Folk Medicines of Bahraich district, Uttar Pradesh". *Ethnobotany,* Vol. 15, No. 1 and 2, 2003, pp. 132-135.

1056. Mandal, S.K. and Basu, S.K. "Ethnobotanical studies among some tribals of Nilgiri district, Tamil Nadu". In Ethnobotany and medicinal plants of Indian Sub-continent, edited by J.K. Maheshwari, Jodhpur, India Scientific Publishers, 2000.

1057. Mandape, Tripali, Joshi, Shailja and Singh, Vir "Use of ethno-phyto medicines in the hills". *Indian Farming*, Vol. 54, No. 4, 2004, pp. 22-23.

1058. Mandelbaum, D. G. "Curing and religion in South Asia" *Journal of the Indian Anthropological Society*, Vol. 5, 1970, pp. 171-186.

1059. Mani, S. B. "From marriage to child conception: An ethnomedical survey in rural Tamil Nadu". In Main Currents in Indian Sociology, edited by Giri Raj Gupta, Vol. 4, 1981, New Delhi, Vikas Publishing House.

1060. Mann, R.S. and Mann, K. "Religious attributes and cure in tribal India". In Tribal health: Socio-Cultural dimentions, edited by Buddhadeb Chaudhuri, New Delhi, Inter India, 1986, pp. 171-184.

1061. Manna, Samita "Role of medicine men in the traditional tribal heritage". *Man in India,* Vol. 83, No. 3-4, 2003, pp. 407-418.

1062. Mao, A. A., "Some symbolic and superstitious botanical folklore about Mao Naga tribe of Manipur, India". In Ethnobotany and medicinal plant of Indian subcontinent, edited by J.K. Maheshwari, Saujanya Books, Jodhpur, 2003, p. 672.

1063. Marrewijk, A.V. "Indigenous knowledge: the proof is in the eating of pudding". *Indigenous knowledge and development Monitor,* Vol. 6, No. 3, 1998, pp. 12-13.

1064. Martin, M. A. "Ethnobotanical aspects of Cannabis in Southeast Asia". In Cannabis and culture edited by V. Rubin, The Hague, Monton, 1975, pp. 63-75.

1065. Mathela, C.S., Kharkwal, H.B. and Joshi, D.N. "Medicinal flora of Pithoragarh district of Uttar Pradesh". *Indian Drug. Pharm, Ind.* Vol. 14, 1979, pp. 34-39

1066. Mathpal, Yoshadhar "Ausadhiprasth". *Himalaya: Man and Nature,* Vol. 14, No. 2-3, 1990, pp. 3-7.

1067. Mathur, A. "Whos ons traditional knowledge?". *Economic and Political Weekly,* Vol. 38, No. 42, pp. 4471-81.

1068. Mathur, P. R. G. "Anthropology of tribal medicine: Disease and curing techniuqes among the tribals of North Wynad (Kerala)". *Man in India,* Vol. 62, No. 3, 1982, pp. 295-312.

1069. Mathur, P. R. G. "Indigenous knowledge, forest ecosystem and native medicine: Vision of biodiversity conservation among the Tribes of Kerala". *Journal of Social Anthropology*, Vol. 6, No. 1-2, 2009, 31-62.

1070. Matpal Himani and Pande, P. C. "Kumaun Himalaya ke Vinayak chetra mai paltu pashuo ki paramparagat chikitsha padhati". Lok Chetna Manch evam Mountain Forum dvara prakashit Parvartika, New Delhi, Vol. 1, 2000, pp. 8-10. [Hindi]

1071. Maurya Umashanker and Srivastava, Shruti "Traditional Indian herbal medicine used as antipyretic, antiulcer, anti-diabetic and anticancer: a review". *International Journal of Research in Pharmacy and Chemistry*, Vol. 1, No. 4, 2011, pp. 1152-1159.

1072. Maya, S, Prameela, Kumari, S. and Menon, V. Sarojini "Ethnobotanical notes on the flora of sacred tanks of Kerala". *Ethnobotany,* Vol. 15, No. 1-2, 2003, pp. 55-59.

1073. Mazars G. "Veterinary medicines in ancient and medieval India". *Studies in History of Science and Medicine,* Vol. 16, No. 1-2, 1999-2000, pp. 27-36.

1074. Mbakogu, Ifeyinwal Annastasia "Forging a link between indigenous communication, effective community social work practice and national development". *Studies of Tribes and Tribals*, Vol. 2, No. 2, 2004, pp. 89-95.

1075. Medhi, B.K. "Ethnomedicine: a study among the Mishings in a rural context". *Bulletin of the Department of Anthropology, Gauhati University*, Vol. 9, 1995, pp. 61—68.

1076. Medhi, B.K. "Folk medicine among the Garos of North-East India". In Tribal studies of North East India, edited by Sarthk Sengupta, New Delhi, Mittal Publicatiosn, 2000, pp. 177-186.

1077. Medhi, B.K. "Use of medicinal plants in the Assamese society". *Bulletin of Folklore Research, Guwahati University,* 2005, pp. 118-130.

1078. Medhi, B.K. and Hasan, Rameeza "Use of plants in the ethno medicinal practices of the Garos of Assam". *Man and Life*, Vol. 29, No. 1&2, 2003, pp. 37-49.

1079. Medhi, Birinchi K. and Hasan, Rameeza "Intangible cultural elements in the ethno-medicinal practices of the Garos of Assam". In Intangible Cultural Heritage of Assam, edited by Kishor. K. Basa and Brinchi K. Medhi, IGRMS, Bhopal and Pratibha Prakashan, Delhi, 2008, pp. 257-270.

1080. Medhi, Birinchi K, and Paul, Bhabatosh "Health and hygiene of the Nahs of Arunachal Pradesh". *Studies of Tribes and Tribals,* Vol. 2, No. 1, 2004, pp. 23-27.

1081. Medhi, Birinchi K. and Saikia, Mahasweta "Indigenous knowledge of the Assamese in the treatment of women's diseases". In Intangible Cultural Heritage of Assam, edited by Kishor. K. Basa and Brinchi K. Medhi, IGRMS, Bhopal and Pratibha Prakashan, Delhi, 2008, pp. 283-291.

1082. Meena, K. L. and Yadav, B. L. "Some ethnomedicinal plant of Southern Rajasthan". *Indian Journal of Traditional Knowledge,* Vol. 9, No. 1, 2010, pp. 169-172.

1083. Mehra, K. L., Kanodia, K. C. and Srivastava, R. N. "Folk uses of plants for adornment in India". Economic Botany, Vol. 29, 1975, pp. 39-46.

1084. Mehrotra, B.N. "Quality control requirements of medicinal plants used in traditional medicines". *Ethnobotany,* Vol. 2, No. 1-2, 1990, pp. 19-24.

1085. Mehrotra, B. N. "Survey of medicinal plants around Kedarnath Shrine of Garhwal Himalaya". Indian Forester, Vol. 105, 1979, pp. 788-801.

1086. Mehrotra, Shanta and Mehrotra, B.N. "Role of traditional and folklore herbals in the development of new drugs". *Ethnobotany,* Vol. 17, No. 1-2, 2005, pp. 104-111.

1087. Mehrotra, Shanta, Rawar, A.K.S. and Singh, H.K. "Standardization of popular ayurvedic adaptogenic preparation 'Chyavanprash' and Ethnobotany of its ingredients". *Ethnobotany,* Vol. 7, No. 1-2, 1995, pp. 1-15.

1088. Mehta, I.S., Joshi, G.C. and Basera, P.S. "The folklore medicinal plants of Talla Johar of Eastern Kumaun Higher Pants of Indian Subcontinent". *Additional Series of Indian Journal of Forestry*, Vol. 3, 1994, pp. 125-133.

1089. Mehta, P.S., Sharma, A.K. and Negi, K.S. "Indigenous knowledge system and sustainable development with particular reference to folklores to Kumaon Himalayan, Uttarakhand". *Indian Journal of Traditional Knowledge,* Vol. 9, No. 3, 2010, pp. 547-550.

1090. Mehta, S.R. "Development of medical sociology in India" *Swasth Hind,* Vol. 29, 1955, pp. 242-247.

1091. Menghani E., Pareek, A., Negi, R.S., and Ojha, C.K. "Antidiabetic potentials of various ethno-medicinal plants of Rajasthan". *Ethnomedicinal Leaflets*, Vol. 14, 2010, pp. 578-583.

1092. Menon, C.K. "Embelia ribes-A medicine for influenza". *Indian forming*. Vol. 45, 1919, pp. 210

1093. Merlin, Mark D. and Kinsela, Georgi M. "Traditional use of turmeric (Curcuma Longa L.) as medicine in Southern Asia and the tropical pacific". *Ethnobotany,* Vol. 17, No. 1-2, 2005, pp. 49-63.

1094. Mhaskar, K.S. and Caius, J.F. "Indian plant remedies used in snake bite". *Indian medical Research Memoirs*, Vol. 19, 1931,

1095. Mibang Tamo and Chaushary, S.K. "Ethnomedicines of the tribes of Arunachal Pradesh". Delhi, Himalayan Publishers, 2003.

1096. Micozzi, Marc S. "Anthropological study of health beliefs, behaviours and outcomes: Traditional folk medicine and ethnopharmacology". *Human Organization*, Vol. 42, No. 4, 1983.

1097. Mishra, A.B. "Pramparagat paudho ka sanrakshan evam patent kaanoon". *Vigyan Pragati*, Vol. 52 No. 12, 2003, pp. 21-24.

1098. Mishra, D.N. "Medicinal plants for the treatment of fever (Jvaracikitsa) in the madhavacikitsd tradition of India". *Indian Journal of Traditional Knbowledge*, Vol. 8, No. 3, 2009, pp. 352-361.

1099. Mishra, D. P. and Sahu, T. R. "Euphorbiaceous plants used in medicine by the tribals of Madhya Pradesh, India". *Journal of Economic and Taxonomic Botany*, Vol. 5, 1984, pp.791-794.

1100. Mishra, Dipak Kumar, Samanta, Godhuli and Mishra, Tapan Kumar "Ethnomedicine of the tribe Kharia of Midnapore district, West Bengal". In Ethnobotany and medicinal plants of Indian Sub-continent, edited by J. K. Maheshwari, Jodhpur, India Scientific Publishers, 2000.

1101. Mishra, Dipak Kumar, Samanta, Godhuli and Mishra, Tapan Kumar "Ethnomedicine of the tribe Kharia of Midnapore district, West Bengal". *Journal of Economic and Taxonomic Botany, Additional Series* Vol. 12, 1996, pp. 329-331.

1102. Mishra Manish "Wild Harvesting and Management of Some Medicinal Plants in the Natural Forest of Central India". *Indian Journal of Fundamental and Applied Life Sciences*, Vol. 1, No. 2, 2011, pp. 90-97.

1103. Mishra, P. K. "Economic development among the Jenu Kurubas". *Man in India*, Vol. 50, 1970, pp. 78-86.

1104. Mishra, P.L."The medicinal plants of Himalaya" . *Himalayan Journal of Sciences*, Vol. 4-5, 1985, pp. 65-80.

1105. Mishra, Prashant Kumar and Ekka, Neeli Rose "An anthropological study of indigenous medicinal practices in a village of Jashpur District, Chhattisgarh". In Traditional Knowledge in Contemporary Societies: Challenges and Apportunities, edited by Kamal K. Misra, IGRMS, Bhopal and Pratibha Prakashan, Delhi, 2007, pp. 231-249.

1106. Mishra, S. P. "Miracles of colour therapy: a guide to drugless system of medicine in health and disease". Calcutta, Firma KLM, 1995, p. 205.

1107. Mishra, T. K., Bhunia, A. and Sahoo, T. K. "Ethnobotany vis-a-vis joint forest management movement of Midnapore (West Bengal), India". *Ethnobotany,* Vol. 9, No. 1-2, 1997, pp. 52-55.

1108. Mishra, Tapan Kumar "Users become managers: Indigenous knowledge and modern forestry". *Economic and Political Weekly,* Vol. 33, No. 6, 1998, pp. 262-263.

1109. Misra, K.K. "Indigenous knowledge, natural resources management and development in a forest-based community of Andhra Pradesh". Report of the major research project submitted to the University Grant Commission, New Delhi. 2004.

1110. Misra, K.K. "Local knowledge, western science and development imperatives, abstract in the proceedings of the 5th Bienniel EASA Conference, Frankfurt (Germany), 1998.

1111. Misra, K.K. and Murthy, M.L.K. (eds.) "Peoples and environment in India". New Delhi, Discovery Publishing House, 2001.

1112. Misra, Kamal K. "Indigenous knowledge, natural resource management and development: Konda Reddi experience". IGRMS, Bhopal and Pratibha Prakashan, Delhi, 2005, p. 299.

1113. Misra, Kamal K. "Traditional knowledge, western science and imperatives of development". *Journal of Indian Anthropological Society*, Vol. 41, No. 2, July 2006, pp. 139-146.

1114. Misra, Kamal K. (ed.) "Traditional knowledge in contemporary societies: Challenges and apportunities". IGRMS, Bhopal and Pratibha Prakashan, Delhi, 2007.

1115. Misra, Kamal K. and Kumar, K. Anil "Ethno- veterinary practices among the Konda reddi of East Godavari district of Andhra Pradesh". *Studies of Tribes and Tribals,* Vol. 2, No. 1, 2004, pp. 37-44.

1116. Misra, Malaya K. "Need for conservation of indigenous medicinal knowledge and the herbs". Journal of Human Ecology, Vol. 10, No. 5-6, 1999, pp. 403-406.

1117. Misra, R.C. "Therapeutic uses of some seeds among the tribals of Gandhamardan range, Orissa". *Indian Journal of Traditional Knowledge,* Vol. 3, No. 1, 2004, pp. 105-115.

1118. Mistry, Nisha, Silori, C.S. and Gupta, L. "Indigenous knowledge on animal healthcare practices in district Kachchh, Gujarat". *Indian Journal of Traditional Knowledge,* Vol. 2, No. 3, 203, pp. 240-254.

1119. Mitalaya, K.D., Bhatt, D.C., Patel, N. K., Didia, S.K. "Herbal medicines used for hair disorders by tribals and rural folk in Gujarat". *Indian Journal of Traditional Knowledge,* Vol. 2, No. 4, 2003, pp. 389-392.

1120. Mittal, K. "Primitive medicine versus modern medicine among the Santals". *Journal of Social Research*, Vol. 12, 1979, pp. 49-54.

1121. Mittre, Vishnu "Wild plants in Indian folk life: A historical perspective". In Glimpses of Indian ethnobotany edited by S. K. Jain, New Delhi, Oxford & IBH, 1981, pp. 37-58.

1122. Moerman, Daniel E. "Anthropology of symbolic healing". *Current Anthropology*, Vol. 20. No. 1, 1979.

1123. Mohammad Sharif "Lok sangeet aur upchar". *Chaumasa*, Vol. 11, No. 35, 1994, pp. 68-74.

1124. Mohammed, Sher, Kasera, Pawan K., Shukla, Jitendra K. "Unexploited plants of potential medicinal value from the Indian Thar desert". *Indian Journal of Natural Products and Resources,* Vol. 3, No. 2, 2004, pp. 69-74.

1125. Mohanty, Jyotsna "Changing scenario of Indigenous knowledge: A study on snake charmers of Orissa". *The Oriental Anthropologist*, Vol. 10, No. 2, 2010, July-Dec. 2010, pp. 221-234.

1126. Mohanty, P.C. "Food habit of a tribal community". *Adibasi,* Vol. 9, 1967, pp. 20-25.

1127. Mohanty, R. B. "Oral and dental healthcare in folklores of Orissa: an ethnobotanical observation". *Ethnobotany,* Vol. 15, No. 1-2, 2003, pp. 125-126.

1128. Mohanty, R.B. and Rout, M.K. "Indigenous rice germplasm and their cultivation technique in folklore of Orissa: an ethnobotanical study". *Ethnobotany,* Vol. 13, No. 1-2, 2001, pp. 24-28.

1129. Mohanty, R.B. Padhy, S.N. and Dash, S.K. "Traditional phytotherapy for diarrhoeal diseases in Ganjan and Phulbani districts of South Orissa, India". *Ethnobotany,* Vol. 8, No. 1-2, 1996, pp. 60-65.

1130. Mohanty, R. B., Dash, B. L. and Dash, N. C. "Ethno-horticultural and olericultural concepts in folklores of Orissa". *Journal of Human Ecology*, Vol. 23, No. 1, 2008, pp. 21-25.

1131. Mohd. Arif Ali "A study of ethnomedicine in a village of Andhra Pradesh". Unpublished M. Phil. Thesis.

1132. Mokat, D.N. and Deokule, S.S. "Plants used as veterinary medicine in Ratnagiri district of Maharashtra". *Ethnobotany,* Vol. 16, No. 1-2, 2004, pp. 131-135.

1133. Molla, H. A. and Roy, B. "Folklore about some medicinal plants from the tribal areas of Jalpaiguri district, West Bengal". *Bulletin of the Botanical Survey of India*, Vol. 26, No. 3-4, 1984, pp. 160-163.

1134. Molla, H. A. and Roy, B. "Some ethnobotanical claims from the Jalpaiguri district of West Bengal". In Ethnobotany and medicinal plants of Indian Sub-continent, edited by J.K. Maheshwari, Jodhpur, India Scientific Publishers, 2000.

1135. Molla, H. A. and Roy, B. "Traditional uses of some medicinal plants by the Rabha tribals of West Bengal", *Journal of Economic and Taxonomic Botany*, Vol. 7, No. 3, 1985, pp. 578-580.

1136. Morris, Brian "Ayurveda and the myth of Indian spirituality". *Man and Life*, Vol. 15, No. 3-4, 1989, pp. 103-122.

1137. Morris, Ramona "Men and snakes". London, Hutchinson, 1965. p. 224.

1138. Muddaiya, R.K., Joshi, G.C. and Pandey, N.K. "Garurbooti Kamaun Himalaya se sarpa dansa ke ek vilakshyan ausadhi evam eska vanaspatik adhyen". Sachitra Ayurved, Vol. 52, November, 1995. [Hindi]

1139. Muddaiya, R.K., Joshi, G.C. & Pandey, N.K. "Status of some valnerable plant species from Ranikhet (Kumoun Himalaya)". Journal of Economic and Taxonomic Botany, Vol. 19, No. 3, 1995, pp. 663-666.

1140. Mudgal, V. and Pal, D.C. "Medicinal plants used by tribals of Mayurbhanj (Orissa)". Bulletin of the Botanical Survey of India, Vol. 22, 1980, pp. 59-62.

1141. Muhuri, Goutam "Professionalisation of traditional medicine of Asia in the 20th century". JREIM, Vol. 10, No. 4, 1991, pp. 29-34.

1142. Mukherjee, Ambarish and Namhata, Debashis "Medicinal plantlore of the tribals of Sundargarh district, Orissa". *Ethnobotany,* Vol. 2, No. 1-2, 1990, pp. 57-60.

1143. Mukherjee, B. "Trends of changes in the Riang culture since independence". Bulletin of Department of Anthropology, Vol. 8, 1959, pp. 103-108.

1144. Mukherjee, B. and others "Traditional medicines". Proceedings of an International Seminar, Calcutta, 7-9, November 1992. New Delhi, Oxford, p. 403.

1145. Mukherjee, D.P. and Nandy, S.K. "Anthropology of tribal health the case of the Asura in Netarhat plateau". In Tribal: Health Socio- Cultural dimentions, edited by B. Chaudhuri, New Delhi, Inter India, 1986, pp. 247-256.

1146. Mukherjee, P.K. and Wahil, A. "Integrated approaches towards drug development from Ayurveda and other systems of medicine". Journal of Ethnopharmacology. Vol. 103, 2006, pp. 25-35.

1147. Mukherjee, Pulok K., Rai, Sujay and Bhattacharya, Sauvik "Marker analysis of polyherbal formulation, triphala - A well known Indian traditional medicine". *Indian Journal of Traditional Knowledge,* Vol. 7, No. 3, 2008, pp. 379-383.

1148. Mukherjee, S.K., Bhujel, R.B., Pradhan, J.P. and Rai, S. "Ethno-medicinal plants of tribals of Bankura district, West Bengal". Journal of Economic and Taxonomic Botany, Vol. 24, No. 2, 2000, pp. 385-394.

1149. Mukherji, B., "Indian indigenous drugs: Need for research", Bulletin of National Institute of Science of India, No. 4, 1955, pp. 1-14.

1150. Mukhopadhyaya, Girindranath "History of Indian medicine: containing notices, biographical and bibliographical of the ayurvedic physicians and their works on medicine (in 3 Vols.)". New Delhi, Oriental Books Reprint Corporation, 1974, p. 868.

1151. Mumgain, S.K. and Rao, R.R. "Some medicinal plants of Pauri Garhwal". Journal of Economic and Taxonomic Botany, Vol. 14, No. 30, 1990, pp. 633-640.

1152. Murmu, Dolly Florence "Plant use among the tribals of Jharkhand". In Tribal health and medicines, edited by A.K. Kalla and P. C. Joshi, New Delhi: Concept Publishing Co., 2004, pp. 351-361.

1153. Murthy, E.N. and others "Piscicidal plants used by Gond tribe of Kawal wildlife sanctuary, Andhra Pradesh, India". Indian Journal of Natural Products and resources, Vol. 1, No. 1, 2010, pp. 97-101.

1154. Murthy, K.S., Sharma, P.C. and Prem Kishore "Tribal remedies for snake bite Orissa". Ancient Science Life, Vol. 6, 1986, pp. 122-123.

1155. Murty, V.V.K. "The tribal people of Rampa and Guden agency of Godavari lower division", Indian Forestry, Vol. 84, 1958, pp. 428-431.

1156. Murugesan, M., Balasubramaniam, V. and Arumugasamy, K. "Ethnomedicinal diversity of Malasars in velliangiri hills, Western Ghats, Tamil Nadu". *Ethnobotany,* Vol. 23, No. 1-2, 2011, pp. 89-99.

1157. Murugesan, M., Balasubramaniam, V. and H. Arthi "Ethno medical knowledge of plants used by Irula tribes, Chengal Combai, the Nilgiris, Tamil Nadu". Ancient Science of Life, Vol. 24, No. 4, 2005, pp. 179-182.

1158. Muthu, C., Ayyanar, M., Raja, N., Ignacimuthu, S. "Medicinal plants used by traditional healers in Kancheepuram District of Tamil Nadu, India". Journal of Ethnobiology and Ethnomedicine, Vol. 2, No. 43, 2006. http://www.ethnobiomed.com/sfx_links?ui=1746-4269-4-22&bibl=B50

1159. Muthukumar, B. "Study on efficacy of siddha drugs (CL and CEN) in rhematoid arthritis". *Indian Journal of Traditional Knowledge,* Vol. 8, No. 3, 2009, pp. 446-448.

1160. Muthukumarasamy, S., Mohan, V.R., Kumaresan, S. and Chelladurai, V. "Herbal medicinal plants used by paliyars to obtain relief from gastro-intestinal complaints". Journal of Economic and Taxonomic Botany, Vol. 27, No. 3, 2003, pp. 711-714.

1161. N., Shiddamallyya, Yasmeen, Azra and Gopakumar, K. "Hundred common forest medicinal plants of Karanataka in primary healthcare". *Indian Journal of Traditional Knowledge,* Vol. 9, No. 1, 2010, pp. 90-95.

1162. Nadkarni, K.M. (ed.) "Indian plants and drugs: With their medical properties and uses". Delhi, Asiatic, 1998, p. 450.

1163. Nag, Ambika, Galav, Praveen and Katewa, S.S. "Indigenous animal healthcare practices from Udaipur district, Rajasthan". *Indian Journal of Traditional Knowledge,* Vol. 6, No. 4, 2007, pp. 583-588.

1164. Nag, Ambika, Galav, Praveen and Katewa, S.S. "Traditional herbal veterinary medicines from Kotda tehsil of Udaipur district (Rajasthan)". *Ethnobotany,* Vol. 21, 1-2, 2009, pp. 103-106.

1165. Nagarajan, S., Jain, H.C. and Aulakh, G.S. "Indigenous of Gujarat". The Eastern Anthropologist. Vol. 4, 1950-51, pp. 42-50.

1166. Nagarajan, S., Jain, H.C. and Aulakh, G.S. "Indigenous plants used in the control of diabetes". In Cultivation and utilisation of medicinal plants, edited by Atal C.K. and B.M. Kapoor, Jammu, Regional Research Lab. CSIR, 1982, pp. 584-604.

1167. Nagendra Prasad, P. and Abraham, Z. "Ethnobotany of Nayadis of North Kerala". Journal of Economic and Taxonomic Botany, Vol. 5, 1984, pp. 41-48.

1168. Nagendra Prasad, P., Singh, A. J. A. Ranjit, Narayanan, L.M. and Natarajan, C. R. "Ethnobotany of the Kanikkars of South Tamil Nadu-I". In Ethnobotany and medicinal plants of Indian Sub-continent, edited by J. K. Maheshwari, Jodhpur, India Scientific Publishers, 2000.

1169. Nagla, Madhu "Sociology of medical profession: a study of medical organizations and profession of medicine in Haryana". Jaipur, Rawat, 1997, p. 268.

1170. Nagnur, Shobha, Channal, Geeta and Channamma, N. "Traditional dairy herd managment practices during pregnancy and calving". Indian Journal of Traditional Knowledge, Vol. 5, No. 2, 2006, pp. 243-244.

1171. Naider, N. Y. "Family planning by tribals". *The Eastern Anthropologist*, Vol. 32, No. 2, 1979, pp. 205-207.

1172. Naidu, B. V. A. Ramarao, Reddi, T. V. V. Seetharami and Prasanthi, S. "Folk herbal remedies for rheimatiod arthritis in Srikakulam district of Andhra Pradesh". *Ethnobotany,* Vol. 20, No. 1-2, 2008, pp. 76-79.

1173. Naik, V. N. "Identification of common Indian medicinal plants". Jodhpur, Scientific Publishers, 2004, p. 150.

1174. Nair, Jeevan "Rich heritage of ancient India". Jaipur, Pointer, 1999, p. 198.

1175. Nair, M.D. "Traditional Chinese medicines: An assessment". *Indian Journal of Traditional Knowledge,* Vol. 2, No. 1, 2003, pp. 7-10.

1176. Nair, N. Vishwanath "Anthropology of tribal health and medicine in forest environment". Kozhikode, KIRTADS, 1995. p. 213.

1177. Nair, N. Vishwanathan "Tribal Health and medicine in Kerala". Kottayam, D.C. Books, 2008, p. 280.

1178. Nair, N. Vishwanathan, "Tribes, healers, medicinal matter and environment". Paper presented at the National workshop on tribal health and medicine in forest environment. Dept. of KIRTADS, Kozhikode, Kerala, 1987.

1179. Nair, R. Madhavan "Tribal healers script a success story" The Hindu, 2 August, 2004.

1180. Nair, V. K. G. "Gender and community medicine". Yojana, Vol. 49, July, 2005, pp. 22-23.

1181. Naithani, B. P. "Medicinal plants of Western Garhwal". Yojana, Vol. 19, 1973, pp. 269-278.

1182. Nambiar, V. P. Krishnan and others "Studies on the medicinal plants of Kerala Forests". Peechi, Kerala Forest Research institute, 1985.

1183. Namhata, D. and Mukherjee, A. "Ethnomedicine in Bankura district, West Bengal". Indian Journal of Applied and Pure Biology, Vol. 3, No. 2, 1988, pp. 53-55.

1184. Nandy, S. K. and Mukherjee, D. P. "Medical Anthropology of a tribal village with special reference to the Asurs, in health and human behaviour". In All Indian Institute of hygiene and public health, edited by B. S. Reddy, 1984.

1185. Nanerjee, Madhulika "Local knowldge for world market: Globalising ayurveda". *Economic and Political Weekly,* Vol. 39, No. 1, 2004, pp. 89-93.

1186. Nanjunda, D.C. and Dinesh, P.T. "Traditional medicine and health commodification: Ethnic people's perception about medicinal plants". Vanyajati, Vol. 59, No. 3, 2011, pp. 32-34.

1187. Nanjunda, D.C., Mahadeviah, V.N., and Roopa, M.C. "Ethno-medicinal plant record of Soliga ethnic group of Karnataka state, India". Vanyajati, Vol. 58, No. 3, 2010, pp. 23-27.

1188. Naqshi, A. R., Baba, M. Y. and Ara, S. "Ethnobotanical studies of Kashmir-Jhelum Valley". Proceedings of Recent advances in Medicinal, Aromatic and Spice Crops in India, New Delhi. 1992, p. 371.

1189. Narayan, Ravi "Towards a people-oriented alternative health care system". Social Action, Vol. 39, No. 3, 1989.

1190. Narayan, S. "Health, forestry and development". In Tribal health: Socio-Cultural dimentions, edited by Buddhadeb Chaudhuri, New Delhi, Inter India, 1986, pp. 325-332.

1191. Narayana Rao, D. "Ayurveda: A survey [Being a brief historical and scientific outline of the indigenous system of medicine from the earliest time to the present day]". Academy of Ayurveda, Delhi, 1950.

1192. Narayanan, A. S. Sankara and Sashiraj, Narmatha "Sholayur Panchayat in Attappady, Kerala: Socio-cultural and ethnobotanical studies on Irula Tribes". Folklore, Vol. 29, No. 4, 1988, pp. 86-90.

1193. Narayanrao, U. B. "Indigenous medicinal specialities". Delhi, Biotech Books, 2003, p. 304.

1194. Naser, Rafiuddin "Traditional plants used as abortifacients in Aurangabad district, Maharashtra". *Ethnobotany,* Vol. 23, No. 1- 2, 2011, pp. 138-140.

1195. Natarajan, D., Balaguru, B. and Nagamurugan, N. "Ethno-medico-botanical survey in the Malligainatham village, Kandarvakottai Taluk, Pudukottai district, Tamil Nadu". *Indian Journal of Traditional Knowledge,* Vol. 9, No. 4, 2010, pp. 768-774.

1196. Natarajan, M. and Govind, Santha "Indigenous agricultural practices among tribal women". *Indian Journal of Traditional Knowledge,* Vol. 5, No. 1, 2006, pp. 118-126.

1197. Nath, Ashish and Maiti, G. G. "Shuktani – a new ethno-medico recipe among the Sylheti Bengali Community of Barak valley, Southern Assam, India". *Indian Journal of Traditional Knowledge,* Vol. 11 No. 1, 2012, pp. 156-160.

1198. Nath, K.K., Deka, P. and Borthakur, S.K. "Traditional remedies of joint diseases in Assam". *Indian Journal of Traditional Knowledge,* Vol. 10, No. 3, 2010, pp. 568-571.

1199. Nath, Subhan C. and Saikia, Nabin "Indigenous knowledge on utility and utilitarian aspects of aquilaria malaccensis lamk in Northeast India". *Indian Journal of Traditional Knowledge,* Vol. 1, No. 1, 2002, pp. 47-58.

1200. Nautiyal S, Maikhuri, R.K., Rao, K.S., Saxena, K. G. "Ethnobotany of the Tolcha Bhotiya tribe of the buffer zone villages in Nanda Devi Biosphere Reserve, India". Journal of Economic and Taxonomic Botany, Vol. 27, No. 1, 2003, pp. 119-142.

1201. Nautiyal, A.R., Nautiyal, M.C. and Purohit, A. N. "Harvesting Herbs-2000, medicinal and aromatic plants – An action plan for Uttarakhand". Bishen Singh Mahendra Pal Singh, DehraDun, 1997.

1202. Nautiyal, B.P. and Nautiyal, S. "Some medicinally important tree species of U.P., Himalaya: Relevance in regional development and ecological security". Journal of Science Research Plant Medicine, Vol. 4, 1983, pp. 14-22.

1203. Nautiyal, S., "Some medicinal plants of Garhwal hills a traditional uses". Journal of Science Research Plant Medicine, Vol. 2, 1981, pp. 12-18.

1204. Navchoo, I. A. and Buth, G.M. "Studies on the medicinal plants used by Gujjar, a backward tribe of Jammu & Kashmir". In Advaces in Plant Science Research, edited by K. C. Sahni, Dehra Dun, Bishen Singh Mahendra Pal Singh, 1994, p. 191.

1205. Nayagam, M. Cyril and Pushparaj, M. S. "Touch me not a medicinal plant of the Nilgiri tribals-a study". In Ethnobotany and medicinal plant of Indian subcontinent, edited by J.K. Maheshwari, Jodhpur, Saujanya Books, 2003, p. 672.

1206. Nayak, A.N. and Babu, B.V. "Tribal Health Problems: An Anthropological Appraisal". *Man in India,* Vol. 83, No. 3, 2003, pp. 301-313.

1207. Nayak, Satish P. and Misra, Malaya K. "Dependence of tribals on forest ecosystem- a case study of Bhogibandha village in Orissa". Journal of Human Ecology, Vol. 2, No. 2, 1991, pp. 135-140.

1208. Nayak, Sobhagini, Behera, Soumit K. and Misra, Malaya K. "Ethno-medico-botanical survey of Kalahandi district of Orissa". *Indian Journal of Traditional Knowledge,* Vol. 3, No. 1, 2004, pp. 72-79.

1209. Nayar, S. L. "Medicinal plants of commercial importance found wild in Uttar Pradesh and their distribution". Journal of Bombay natural History Society, Vol. 61, 1964, pp. 651-661.

1210. Nazarea, Virginia D. "Local Knowledge and Memory in Biodiversity Conservation". Annual Review of Anthropology, Vol. 35, 2006, pp. 317-335.

1211. Nazarudeen, A., Seeni, S., Koshy, K.C. & Pushpangadan, P. "Folk plants of food, medicine, adornment and repellent used by the Paniyar community in North Kerala". In Ethnobotany and medicinal plants of Indian Sub-continent, edited by J.K. Maheshwari, Jodhpur, India Scientific Publishers, 2000.

1212. Negi, Chandra S. and Palyal, Veerendra S. "Traditional uses of animal and animal products in medicine and rituals by the Shoka tribes of district Pithoragarh, Uttaranchal, India". Studies on Ethno-Medicine, Vol. 1, No. 1, 2007, pp. 47-54.

1213. Negi, Chandra Singh "Socio-cultural and ethnobotanical value of a sacred forest, Thal Ke Dhar, central Himalaya". *Indian Journal of Traditional Knowledge,* Vol. 4, No. 2, 2005, pp. 190-198.

1214. Negi, K.S. and Gaur, R.D. "A contribution to the Indian wild edible fruits of U.P. hills". Bulletin of Botanical Survey of India, Vol. 33, No. 1-4, 1991, pp. 233-266.

1215. Negi, K. S. and Gaur, R. D. "Little known wild Allium species in the Uttar Pradesh hills". Mountain Research and Development, Vol. 11, No. 2, 1991, pp. 162-164.

1216. Negi, K.S. and Pant, K.C. "Less known wild species of Allium Linn (Amaryllidaceae) form mountainous region of India". Economic Botany, Vol. 46, No. 1, 1992, pp. 112-116.

1217. Negi, K.S. and Pant, K.C. "Notes on Ethnobotany of the Gangwal: a tribe of Garhwal Himalaya". *Ethnobotany,* Vol. 2, No. 1-2, 1990, pp. 81-85.

1218. Negi, K.S., Gaur, R.D. and Tiwari, J.K. "Ethnobotanical notes on the Flora of Har-Ki-Doon (district Uttarkashi), Garhwal Himalaya, Uttar Pradesh, India". *Ethnobotany,* Vol. 11, No. 1-2, 1999, pp. 9-17.

1219. Negi, K.S., Tiwari, J.K. & Gaur, R. D. "Economic importance of some common trees in Garhwal Himalaya: An ethnobotanical study". Indian Journal of Forestry, Vol. 8, No. 4, 1985, pp. 276-289.

1220. Negi, K.S., Tiwari, J.K. and Gaur, R.D. "Ethnobotanical importance of some trees in Garhwal Himalayas". Journal of Indian Botanical Society, Vol. 61 (Suppl.), 1985, p. 32.

1221. Negi, K.S., Tiwari, J.K. and Gaur, R.D. "Notes on Ethnobotany of five districts of Garhwal Himalaya, Uttar Pradesh, India". *Ethnobotany,* Vol. 5, No. 1-2, 1993, pp. 73-81.

1222. Negi, Roshan Singh, Sharma, Kailash Chand and Sharma, Manju "Micropropagation and anatomical comparision of in vivo and in vitro developed shoot and root in cassia auriculata L.- A medicinally important plant". Indian Journal of Fundamental and Applied Life Sciences, Vol. 1, No. 1, 2011, pp. 21-29.

1223. Negi, Vikram S., Maikhuri, R.K. and Vashishtra, D.P. "Traditional healthcare practices among the villages of Rawain valley, Uttarkashi, Uttarakhand, India". *Indian*

Journal of Traditional Knowledge, Vol. 10, No. 3, 2011, pp. 533-537.

1224. Nehru, Jawaharlal, "The Tribal folk". In The Adivasis, New Delhi, Director, publications division, Government of India. 1960.

1225. Nepali, Gopal Singh "Newars: An Ethno-Sociology study of a Himalayan community". Bombay, United Asia Publications, 1965, p. 476.

1226. Nesamony, S. "Oushadha sasyangal". Thiruvanatpuram, State Institute of Language, 1989, p. 514. [Malayalam]

1227. Neumann, A. K. "Role of indigenous medicine practitioner in two areas of India: Report of a study". Social sciences and medicine, Vol. 5, 1971, pp. 141-142.

1228. Nichter, Mark "Healing in the modern state: political ecology of health in India". Traditional Medicine, Shamanism, and Science in Asian Societies, 2001, pp. 85-106.

1229. Nichter, Mark "Towards a culturally responsive rural health care delivery system in India". In Main currents in Indian Sociology, Vol.- IV, edited by Giriraj Gupta New Delhi, Vikas Publishing House Pvt. Ltd, 1981, pp. 223-236.

1230. Nirala, Sanjay Kumar and Bhagat, Anjani "Bhaina Janjati aur vanausadhi: ek Manav Sastriya Addhyan". Vanyajati, Vol. 57, No. 3, 2009, pp. 46-54.

1231. Nirmal Kumar J. I. and others "Studies on plant species used by tribal communities of Saputara and Purna forests, Dangs district, Gujarat". *Indian Journal of Traditional Knowledge,* Vol. 6, No. 2, 2007, pp. 368-374.

1232. Nirmale, V.H., Sontakki, B.S. and Biradar, R.S. "Use of indigenous knowledge by coastal fisher folk of Mumbai district in Maharashtra". *Indian Journal of Traditional Knowledge,* Vol. 6, No. 2, 2007, pp. 378-382.

1233. Nirmale, Vivek H., Sontakki, Bharat S. and Biradar, R. S. "Assessment of indigenous knowledge of coastal fisher folk of greater Mumbai and Sindhudurg districts of Maharashtra". *Indian Journal of Traditional Knowledge,* Vol. 3, No. 1, 2004, pp. 27-36.

1234. Nisteswar, K. "Project profiles of herbal and traditional medicine based integrated health system in tribal areas of Andhra Pradesh". Indian Medicine (Vijayawada), Vol. 4, No. 2, 1992, pp. 2-6.

1235. Noumi, Emmanuel "Ethno-medico-botanical survey of medicinal plants used in the treatment of asthma in the Nkongsamba region, Cameroon". *Indian Journal of Traditional Knowledge,* Vol. 9, No. 3, 2009, pp. 491-495.

1236. O'Connor B. B. "Healing traditions: Alternative medicine and the health Profession". University of Pennsylvania Press, Philadelphia, Pennsylvania. 1995.

1237. Obeyesekere, Gananath "The cultural background of sinhalese medicine". Journal of Indian Anthropological Society, Vol. 4, No. 1-2, 1969, pp. 117-139.

1238. Oinam, Santaram S., Kuniyal, Jagdish C. and Rawat, Yashwant S, "Indigenous knowledge application for conservation of Bio- resource in the cold desert of the Northwestern Himalaya". Journal of Social Anthropology, Vol. 6, No. 1-2, 2009, pp. 75-86.

1239. Olatokun, Wole Michael "Indigenous knowledge of traditional medical practitioners in the treatment of sickle cell anemia". *Indian Journal of Traditional Knowledge,* Vol. 9, No.1, 2010, pp. 119-125.

1240. Opler, M. E. "Cultural definition of illness in village India". Human Organiztion, Vol. 22, No. 1, 1963, pp. 32-35.

1241. Padhy, S. N., Dash, S. K. and Mohapatra, Ratnaprava "The Vedic Soma plant, how much Ethnobotanical?: an introspective review". *Ethnobotany,* Vol. 13, No. 1-2, 2001, pp. 45-49.

1242. Paharai, "Travails of Traditional medicine". In History of Medicine in India: The Medical encounter, edited by Chittabrata Palit and Achintya Dutta, Delhi, Kalpaz Publications, 2005, pp. 219-234.

1243. Pai, D.N. and Entructur, M.I. "Health of the rural adivasis in India". Journal of Medical Science, Vol. 18, No. 3, 1964, pp. 716.

1244. Painuli, R.M. and Maheshwari, J.K. "Some interesting ethnomedicinal plants used by Sahariya tribe of Madhya Pradesh". In Ethnobotany and medicinal plants of Indian sub-continent, edited by J. K. Maheshwari, Jodhpur, India Scientific Publishers, 2000.

1245. Pal, D.C. "Magico-religious beliefs about plants among adibasis of Bihar". Folklore, Vol. 13, No. 12, 1972, pp. 479-493.

1246. Pal, D.C. "Observation on folklore about plants in venterinary medicine in Bengal, Orissa and Bihar". Bulletin of the Botanical Survey of India, Vol. 22, 1980, pp. 96-99.

1247. Pal, D.C. "Plants used in treatment of cattle and birds among tribal of eastern India". In Glimpses of Indian Ethnobotany, edited by S. K. Jain, New Delhi: Oxford & IBH, 1981, pp. 245-257.

1248. Pal, D.C. "Tribal folk lore about some plants associated with eye treatment". Folklore, Vol. 14, No. 12, 1973, pp. 446-447.

1249. Pal, D.C. and Banerjee, D.K. "A note on the plants used by the tribals in India for hair and scalp preparation". Folklore, Vol. 18, No. 1, 1977, pp. 1-5.

1250. Pal, D. C. and Banerjee, D. K. "Plants used by the tribal people in Orissa for hair and scalp preparation". Adibasi, Vol. 15, No. 1-4, 1974, pp. 28-32.

1251. Pal, D.C. and Banerjee, D.K. "Some less known plant foods among the tribals of Andhra Pradesh and Orissa State". Bulletin of the Botanical Survey of India, Vol. 13, 1971, pp. 221-223.

1252. Pal, D.C. and Guha, A. "Some Tribal Habit about Honey". Folklore, Vol. 22, No. 5, 1981, pp. 107-108.

1253. Pal, D.C. and Jain, S. K. "Notes on Lodha medicine in Midnapur district W. B. India". Economic Botany, Vol. 43, 1989, pp. 464-470.

1254. Pal, D.C. and Jain, S. K. "Tribal Medicine". Naya Prokash, Culcutta, 1998, p. 317.

1255. Pal, D.C. and Saren, A. M. "Indian Plants and connected Folklore: an account of a few plants in tribal life". Folklore, Vol. 27, No. 9, 1986, pp. 198-200.

1256. Pal, D.C., Bhattacharjee, A.K. and Guha, A. "Perspectives of tribal concept about disease in traditional system". In Tribal health: Socio-Cultural dimentions, edited by

Buddhadeb Chaudhuri, New Delhi, Inter India, 1986, pp. 167-170.

1257. Pal, Sanjoy Kumar "Complementary and alternative medicine: An overview". Current Science, Vol. 82, No. 5, 2002, pp. 518-524.

1258. Palekar, R.P. "Ethno-medical traditions of Thakur tribals of Karjat, Maharashtra". Ancient Science of Life, Vol. 12, No. 3/4, 1993, pp. 388-393.

1259. Palit, Chittabrata and Dutta, Achintya Kumar (eds.) "History of medicine in India: the medical encounter". Delhi, Kalpaz Publications, 2005. p. 355.

1260. Paliwal, G. S. and Badoni, A. K. "Ethnobotany of hill tribes of Uttarkashi, II. Medicinal plants". Journal of Economic and Taxonomic Botany, Vol. 14, 1990, pp. 421-442.

1261. Panda S. "Plant use-a recent perspective from Eastern Himalayas". In Ethnobotany and medicinal plants of Indian Sub-continent, edited by J. K. Maheshwari, Jodhpur, India Scientific Publishers, 2000.

1262. Panda, Ashok Kumar and Mishra, Sangram "Some belief, practices and prospects of folk healers of Sikkim". *Indian Journal of Traditional Knowledge,* Vol. 11, No. 2, 2012, pp. 369-373.

1263. Panda, Basant Kumar "Some ethnomedicinal plants of Karlapat Reserve Forest, district Kalahandi, Orissa". *Ethnobotany,* Vol. 19, No. 1&2, 2007, pp. 134-136.

1264. Panda, N.C. "Folk Medicine in Western Orissa: some Tribal and Folk Cultural practices". Folklore, Vol. 28, No. 12, 1987, pp. 289-294.

1265. Panda, P. C. and Das, P. "Medicinal plant-lore of the tribals of Baliguda sub-division, Phulbani district, Orissa". In Ethnobotany and medicinal plant of Indian subcontinent, edited by J.K. Maheshwari, Saujanya Books, Jodhpur, 2003, p. 672.

1266. Panda, Tribhubana, Panigrahi, Srikanta K. and Padhy, Rabindra N. "A sustainable use of phytodiversity by the Kandha tribe of Orissa". *Indian Journal of Traditional Knowledge,* Vol. 4, No. 2, 2005, pp. 173-178.

1267. Pande, B.C., Datt, Bhaskar & Pande, P.C. "Notes on the ethnomedicinal aspect of some common Pteridophytes of Almora district of Kumaun Himalaya (Uttaranchal)". *Ethnobotany,* 12, 2000, pp. 56-59.

1268. Pande, Deep Chandra and Pande, P.C. "Kumaun Himalaya ka lok vanshpati vigyan (in Hindi)". In Yug Yugeen Uttaranchal edited by C. M. Agarwal, Indian Publishers Distributes, New Delhi. pp 175-193, 2001.

1269. Pande, G. "Ganjiyari –a traditional herbal drug of Uttarakhand Himalayas". Sachitra Ayurved, Vol. 46, 1993, pp. 118-120.

1270. Pande, G. "Kubjak in Uttarakhand Himalaya: A traditional medicinal plants". Sachitra Ayurved, Vol. 46, 1994, pp. 571-573.

1271. Pande, N.K. "Drug potential and conservation notion of medicinal plants of Western Himalaya". Journal of Research and Education in Indian Medicine, Vol. 10, 1991, pp. 29-40.

1272. Pande, N. K. and others "Medicinal plants of Kumaun Himalaya and strategies for conservation". In Himalayan Biodiversity: Conservation Strategies edited by U. Dhar, Gyanodaya Prakashan, Nainital, 1993.

1273. Pande, N. K., Joshi, G. C. & Uniyal, M. R. "Conservation inventory of high altitude medicinal plants of Western Himalaya used in Indian system of medicine". Conference of Pharmacology and Symposium on Herbal Drugs, (New Delhi), 1994, p. 14.

1274. Pande, P.C. "Prakrity". In Soldier edited by C. M. Agrwal, Indian Publishers Distributors, New Delhi, 2000, pp: 159-166.

1275. Pande, P.C. and Joshi, G.C. "Cultivated plants of Kumaun Himalaya used for medicinal purpose". In Himalayan medicinal plants: Potential and prospects edited by S.S. Samant, U. Dhar and L.M.S. Palni, Gyanodaya Prakasan, Nainital, 2001, pp. 117-125.

1276. Pande, P.C. and Joshi, Pramila "Food and Food Habits of Kumaunies (Western Himalaya)". In Man Culture & Society in the Kumaun Himalayas edited by C. M. Agrwal, Sri Almora Book Depot, Almora, 1996, pp. 163-179.

1277. Pande, P.C. and Mahesh Chandra "Kumaun ke Bageshwar chetra mai pashuo ki paramparik chikitsha paddathi". In Uttaranchal Ke Sanchal Se edited by C.M. Agrwal, Indian Publishers, New Delhi, 2001, pp. 19-40. [Hindi]

1278. Pande, P. C. and Mamgai, Laxmi "Kumaun ke Mashi ke najdeek Bhumka Pani Chhetra mai parmparagat pashu chikitsha". Syvadhin Praja, Vol. 8, No. 4, 2001. pp. 12-13. [Hindi]

1279. Pande, P. C. and Pande, H. C. "Traditional Usage of 'Urad' (Vigna mungo) in Kumaon Himalaya, Uttaranchal". *Ethnobotany,* Vol. 16, No. 1-2, 2004, pp. 96-98.

1280. Pande, P.C. and Pangtey, Y.P.S. "Studies on the ethnobotany- I. On some less known edible and economic ferns of Kumaun region of Western Himalaya". Journal of Economic and Taxonomic Botany, Vol. 11, No.1, 1987, pp. 139-148.

1281. Pande, P.C., Joshi, G.C. and Kandpal, M.M. "Ethnobotany of Kumaun Himalayas". In Himalayas: Environment, resources and development edited by N.K. Sah, S.D. Bhatt and R.K. Pande, Shree Almora Book Depot, Almora, 1989, pp. 255-294.

1282. Pande, P.C., Joshi, Pramila and Pande, H.C. "Studies on the ethnobotany II. On some less known medicinal and economic ferns of Kumaun region of Western Himalaya". In Current Research in Plant Science edited by T.A. Sharma, S.S. saini, M. L. Trivedi and M. Sharma, Bishen Singh and Mahendra Pal Singh, Dehra Dun. 1984, pp. 135-137.

1283. Pande, P.C., Tiwari, L. and Pande, H.C. "Folk medicine and Aromatic plants of Uttraranchal Himalay". Bishen Singh Mahendrapal Singh, Dehradun, 2006.

1284. Pandey, Ashok K., Bora, H.R. & Deka, S.C. "An ethno-medico-botanical study of Golaghat district, Assam: native plant remedies for jaundice". In Ethnobotany and medicinal plants of Indian Sub-continent, edited by J.K. Maheshwari, Jodhpur, India Scientific Publishers, 2000.

1285. Pandey, G and Joshi, G. C. "Gujkarul (Ramkarela) Uttar Pradesh ki Himalaya shetra ka aprisadha sak". Sachitra Ayurved, March 1992, pp. 581-582. [Hindi)]

1286. Pandey, G., Joshi, G.C., Pandey, N.K. and Tewari, K.C. "Ethnobotanical Studies on the medicinal flora of Tarikhet block (Kamaun Himalaya) district. Almora, U.P. Part-IV". Aryavaidyan, Vol. 8, No. 3, 1995, pp. 159-164.

1287. Pandey, G., Joshi, G.C., Pandey, N.K. and Tewari, K.C. "Ethnobotanical Studies on the medicinal flora of Tarikhet block (Kumaun Himalaya) district Almora, U.P. Part II". Aryavaidyan, Vol. 8, No. 1, 1994, pp. 40-46.

1288. Pandey, G., Joshi, G.C., Pandey, N.K. and Tewari, K.C. "Ethnobotanical studies on the medicinal flora of Tarikhet block (Kumaun Himalaya) district Almora, U.P. Part-I". Ayurvaidyan, Vol. 7, No. 4, 1994, pp. 212-223.

1289. Pandey, G., Joshi, G.C., Pandey, N.K. and Tewari, K.C. "Ethnobotanical studies on the medicinal flora of Tarikhet block (Kamaun Himalaya) district Almora, U.P. Part-III". Aryavaidyan, Vol. 8, No, 2. 1994, pp. 74-79.

1290. Pandey, G., Singh, V.K. and Bhatnagar, L.S. "New records to the medical efficacy claims of certain plants recorded from Guntour forest circle, M. P. -A preliminary contribution". Bulletin of Medico-ethno-botanical Research, Vol. 2, 1981, pp. 303-315.

1291. Pandey, Gyanendra "Dravyaguna Vijnana=Materia Medica-Vegetable Drugs: [English-Sanskrit]". Varanasi, Krishnadas Academy, 1998, p. 943.

1292. Pandey, Gyanendra "System of plant nomenclature in Ayurveda". Varanasi, Chowkhamba Sanskrit Series Office, 1997, p. 603.

1293. Pandey, Hari Prakash "Seed Oil of Butea Monosperma: a traditional sexual toner and contraceptive". *Ethnobotany,* Vol. 13, No. 1-2, 2001, pp. 118-120.

1294. Pandey, Indu Bhushan "Some Traditional Herbal Home Remedies used in and around Kanpur city (Uttar Pradesh), India". *Ethnobotany,* Vol. 15, No. 1-2, 2003, pp. 129-131.

1295. Pandey, Keya "An ethnobotanical approach to the vanishing tribe Raji". Proceedings of 7th Indian Science Congress, Pune, 3-7, Jan. 2000.

1296. Pandey, Keya and Pandey, Suresh "Indigenous medicines of raji tribes of Uttarakhand". *Indian Journal of Traditional Knowledge,* Vol. 9, No. 1, 2010, pp. 131-133.

1297. Pandey, Keya and Tiwari, S. P. "Studies on ethnobotanical approach tof the vanishing tribe Raji". Journal of Economic and Taxonomic Botany, Vol. 27, No. 4, 2003, pp. 947-955.

1298. Pandey, M.J., Joshi, G.C. & Pandey, G. "Athervedkta ausadhi parichaya". Sachitra Ayurved, March 1993, pp. 538-540. [Hindi]

1299. Pandey, Shivendra Kumar "Krashi aur ausadhi chhetra me gobar va mootra ka arthik mahattva".Yojana, Vol. 44, No. 12, 2001, pp. 7-12. [Hindi]

1300. Pandey, V. N. "Primary health care application and utilisation of Ayurvedic/traditional/tribal system of medicine -A view point". Journal of Research and Education in Indian Medicine, Vol. 8, No. 4, 1989, pp. 1-16.

1301. Pandit, Apoorvaa "Indigenous technological knowledge and practices of the tribal people in Maharashtra". Journal of Human ecology, Vol. 12, No. 6, 2001, pp. 469-472.

1302. Pangtey, Y. P. S., Samant, S. S. and Rawat, G. S. "Ethnobotanical notes on Bhotia tribes of Kumaun Himalaya". Indian Journal of Forestry, Vol. 12, No. 2, 1989, pp. 191-196.

1303. Panigrahi, Nilakantha "Ethnomedicine among the Gonds of Orissa". In Tribal demography in India edited by Rabindra Nath Pati and Laltendu Jagatdeb, New Delhi, Ashish Publishing House, 1991, pp. 20-37.

1304. Panikkar, K. M. "Indigenous Medicine and Cultural hegemony: A Study of Revitalisation movement in Kerala". Aryavaidyan, Vol. 8, No. 1, 1994, pp. 28-39.

1305. Pant, G. and Tiwari, S. D. "Bryophytes and mankind". *Ethnobotany,* Vol. 2, No.1-2, 1990, pp. 97-103.

1306. Pant, G. and Tiwari, S. D. "Various human uses of Bryophytes in the Kumaun region of North West Himalaya". Bryologist, Vol. 92, 1989 pp. 120-122.

1307. Pant, S. C. and Pande, G. "Ethnobotanical studies on medicinal flora of Tharu tribal pokets in Kumaun region in Uttar Pradesh". Seminar on Research Ayurveda and Shiddha, CCRAS, New Delhi, 20-22, March, 1995. p. 51.

1308. Paochunbou, K. "Tribal Medicine". (http://e-pao.net/ epSubPage Extractor.asp? src=education. Health_Issue. Tribal_Medicine).

1309. Parabia, Minoo and Pathak, Smita "Use of herbal resources in primary healthcare and the knowledge feedback mechanism as an interactive system for tribal". *Ethnobotany,* Vol. 20, No. 1-2, 2008, pp. 106-110.

1310. Paranjpe, Prakash "Indian medicinal plants: Forgotten healers a guide to ayurvedic herbal medicine". Delhi, Chaukhamba Sanskrit Pratishthan, 2001, p. 316.

1311. Parihar, Pradeep and Parihar, Leena "Some pteridophytes of medicinal importance from Rajasthan". Indian Journal of Natural Products and Resources, Vol. 5, No. 4, 2006, p. 297-301.

1312. Parinitha, M., Harish, G. U. and Vivek, N. C. "Ethno-botanical wealth of Bhadra wild life sanctuary in Karnataka". *Indian Journal of Traditional Knowledge,* Vol. 3, No. 1, 2004, pp. 37-50.

1313. Park, John Everett "Textbook of preventive and social medicine: a treatise on community health". Banarsidas Bhanot, 1972, p. 716.

1314. Parkash, Vipin and Aggarwal, Ashok "Traditioanl uses of ethnomedicinal plants of lower foot- hills of Himachal Pradesh-I". *Indian Journal of Traditional Knowledge,* Vol. 9, No. 3, 2009, pp. 519-521.

1315. Parle, Milind and Bansal, Nitin "Herbal Medicines: Are they safe?". Indian Journal of Natural Products and Resources, Vol. 5, No. 1, 2006, pp. 6-14.

1316. Patel, N.B., Sidana, B.S. and Jain, B.K. "Tribal Artefacts of Dholwani Forest of Sabarkantha: Gujrat". *Ethnobotany,* Vol. 15, No. 1-2, 2003 pp. 40-43.

1317. Patel, Vibha J. "Shamans of Nagaland". The India Magazine, Vol. 14, No. 6, 1994, pp. 18-27.

1318. Pathak, N.N. and Karnick, C.R. "New folk-lore medicines from Sudh-Mahadeo region of Himalayas". Nagarjun Vol. 23, No. 11, 1980, pp. 242-245.

1319. Pathak, N. N. and Karnick, C. R. "Newer observations on the crude drug termed as 'Tikta' from Laddak (Himalayas) region". Nagarjun, Vol. 25, No. 1, 1981, pp. 4-6.

1320. Pathak, R.D. "Intellegence and Intrest among Mizo Students of Shillong: (A Study in Ethno-Psychology)".

Bulletin of the Anthropological Survey of India, Vol. 28, No. 1-2, 1979. pp. 1-20.

1321. Pati, R.N. "Ethno-medicinal practices and sustainable development: sensitive issues of economic transformation in Chhattisgarh". Journal of the Indian Anthropological Society, Vol. 40, No. 1, 2005, pp. 65-74.

1322. Patil, D.A. "Origin of Medicine vis-a-vis Doctrine of Signatures". *Ethnobotany,* Vol. 16, No. 1-2, 2004, pp. 52-58.

1323. Patil, H.M. and Bhaskar, V.V. "Medicinal knowledge system of tribals of Nandurbar district, Maharashtra". *Indian Journal of Traditional Knowledge,* Vol. 5, No. 3, 2006, pp. 327-330.

1324. Patil, H.M. and Bhaskar, V.V. "Medicinal uses of plants by tribal medicine men of Nandurbar district in Maharashtra". Indian Journal of Natural Products and Resources, Vol. 5, No. 2, 2006, pp. 125-130.

1325. Patil, Jayshri U., Biradar, S.D. "Folkloric medicinal plants of Hingoli district, Maharashtra". Indian Journal of Natural Products and Resources, Vol. 2, No. 1, 2011, pp. 97-101.

1326. Patil, M.V. and Patil, D.A. "Ethnomedicinal practices of Nasik District, Maharashtra". *Indian Journal of Traditional Knowledge,* Vol. 4, No. 3, 2005, pp. 287-290.

1327. Patil, M.V., and Patil, D.A. "Some herbal remedies used by the tribals of Nasik district, Maharashtra". Indian Journal of Natural Products and Resources, Vol. 6, No. 2, 2007, pp. 152-157.

1328. Patil, S.H. "Ethno-medico-zoological studies on Nandubar district of Maharashtra". *Indian Journal of Traditional Knowledge,* Vol. 2, No. 3, 2003, pp. 297-299.

1329. Patil, S.H. and Merat, Manoj M. "Ethnoveterinary practices in Satpudas of Nandurbar district of Maharashtra". *Ethnobotany,* Vol. 15, No. 1-2, 2003, pp. 103-106.

1330. Patil, S.H. and Yadav, S.S. "Traditional medicinal plants of Satpuda, Nandurbar district Maharashtra state". Indian Forester, Vol. 129, No. 11, 2003, pp. 1379-1385.

1331. Patil, S.L. and Patil, D.A. "Ethnomedicinal plants of Dhule district, Maharashtra". Natural Product Radiance, Vol. 6, No. 2, 2007, pp. 148-151.

1332. Patnaik, Chranjibi, Reddy, C., Das, Rasmita and Reddy, Manikya "Traditional medicinal practices among the tribal people of Malkangiri district Orissa, India". Indian Journal of Natural Product Rediance, Vol. 6, No. 5, 2007, pp. 430-435.

1333. Patra, Kartik Chand, Kumar, K. Jayaram and Suresh, P. "Standardization of a polyherbal siddha formulation, Amukkara Choornam". *Indian Journal of Traditional Knowledge,* Vol. 8, No. 3, 2009, pp. 449-452.

1334. Patra, Kartik Chandra and others "Traditional approaches towards standardization of herbal medicines-A review". Journal of Pharmaceutical Science and Technology, Vol. 2, No. 11, 2010, pp. 372-379.

1335. Patrick, O. E. "Herbal Medicines: Challenges". Tropical Journal Pharmaceutical Research, Vol. 1, No. 2, 2002, pp. 53-54.

1336. Pattanaik, Chiranjibi, Dhal, N.K., Rout, N.C. and Reddy, Ch. Sudhakar "Folk medicinal plants of Satkosia Gorge Sanctuary, Orissa, India". In Traditional Knowledge in Contemporary Societies: Challenges and Apportunities, edited by Kamal K. Misra and K.K. Basa, IGRMS, Bhopal and Pratibha Prakashan, Delhi, 2007, pp. 223-230.

1337. Pattanaik, Debasish and Jha, Munmun "Knowledge and identity among the indigenous people". The Oriental Anthropologist, Vol. 7, No. 2, 2007, pp. 199-212.

1338. Patwardhan, Bhushan, Chopra, Arvind and Vaidya, Ashok D. B. "Herbal remedies and the bias against Ayurveda". Current Science, Vol. 84, No. 9, 2003, pp. 1165-1166.

1339. Patwardhan, Bhushan, Joglekar, Vishnu and Pathak, Namyata "Vaidya-scientists: Catalysing Ayurveda renaissance". Current Science, Vol. 100, No. 4, 2011, pp. 476-483.

1340. Patwardhan, Bhushan, Vaidya, Ashok D.B. and Chorghade, Mukund "Ayurveda and natural products drug discovery". Current Science, Vol. 86, No. 6, 2004, pp. 789-799.

1341. Paul, D.C. and Saren, A.M. "Unknown local names and uses of some Indian medicinal plants: an appraisal". Folklore, Vol. 32, No. 5-6, 1991, pp. 91-93.

1342. Paul, K. "Tribal Health and Development: Some Socio-Cultural Dimensions". The Oriental Anthropologist, Vol. 5, No. 2, 2005, pp. 257-268.

1343. Paul, S. R. "Medicinal plants of Netarhat, Bihar (India)". Quarterly Journal of Crude Drug Research, Vol. 15, 1977, pp. 79-97.

1344. Paul, T. K. and Mudgal, V. "Unreported medicinal uses of some plants recorded from the tribals of Koraput (Orissa)". Bulletin of Botanical Survey of India, Vol. 27, 1985, pp. 69-71.

1345. Pawar, Shubhangi and Patil, D. A. "Herbal Folk Remedies for Urinogenital Complaints in Jalgaon district of Maharashtra". *Ethnobotany,* Vol. 16, No. 1-2, 2004, pp. 86-90.

1346. Pawar, Shubhangi and Patil, D.A. "Obervations on folkloric medicinal plants of Jalgaon district, Maharashtra". *Indian Journal of Traditional Knowledge,* Vol. 3, No. 4, 2004, pp. 437-441.

1347. Pawar, Shubhangi, Patil, M.V. and Patil, D.A. "Fish Stupefying Plants used by Tribals of North Maharashtra". *Ethnobotany,* Vol. 16, No. 1-2, 2004, pp. 136-138.

1348. Payyappallimana, Unnikrishnan "From Rio to Reality: A Case Study of Bio-prospecting Local Health Knowledge in Kani Tribal Community of Kerala, India". Amsterdam Master's in Medical Anthropology (AMMA) Medical Anthropology Unit, Faculty of Social and Behavioural Sciences, University of Amsterdam The Netherlands, Amsterdam, August 2000.

1349. Pei, S. J. "Ethnobotanical approaches of traditional medicine studies: some experiences from Asia". Pharmaceutical Biology, Vol. 39, 2001, pp. 74-79.

1350. Perez, Joseph Marti I. "Encountering the irrational: Some reflections on folk healers". Folklore, Vol. 99, No. 2, 1988, pp. 178-185.

1351. Perumal Samy, R. and Ignacimuthu, S. "Antibacterial activity of some folklore medicinal plants used by tribals in Western Ghats of India". Journal of Ethnopharmacology Vol. 69, 2000, pp. 63-71.

1352. Phartiyal, P. C. "Uttaranchal mai jari bootiyo ke kastkar avam sansthan nideshika". Central Development Studies, U.P. Academy Administration, Nainital, 1998. [Hindi]

1353. Pinto, Sarah "Development without Institutions: Ersatz Medicine and the Politics of Everyday Life in Rural North India". Cultural Anthropology, Vol. 19, No. 3, 2004, pp. 337-364.

1354. Polunin, Ivan. "Some Characteristics of Tribal People". In Health and disease in tribal societies, CIBA foundation symposium 49, New York, Elsevier-Excerpta Medica, 1977.

1355. Posey, D. and others "Indigenous Peoples, Traditional Technologies and Equitable Benefit Sharing: International Instruments for the Protection of Community Intellectual Property and Traditional Resource Rights". Oxford, Working Group on Traditional Resource Rights. 1994.

1356. Prabhakar, Amit Kumar and Roy, S.P. "Ethno-medicinal uses of some shell fishes by people of Kosi River Basin of North-Bihar, India". Studies on ethno-medicine, Vol. 3, No. 1, 2009, pp. 1-4.

1357. Prachi, Chauhan, N. and Kumar, D. "Medicinal plants muzaffarnagar district used in treatment of urinary tract and kidney stones". *Indian Journal of Traditional Knowledge,* Vol. 8, No. 2, 2009, pp. 191-195.

1358. Pradhan, Bharat K. and Badola, Hemant K. "Ethnomedicinal plant use by Lepcha tribe of Dzongu valley, bordering Khangchendzonga Biosphere Reserve, in North Sikkim, India" Journal of Ethnobiology and Ethnomedicine, Vol. 4, No. 22, 2008.

1359. Prajapati, Narayan Das "Handbook of medicinal plants: A complete source book". Jodhpur, Agrobios India, 2003, p. 158.

1360. Prakash, H. M. and Krishnappa, M. "People's knowledge on medicinal plants in Sringeri taluk, Karnataka". *Indian Journal of Traditional Knowledge,* Vol. 5, No. 3, 2006, pp. 353-357.

1361. Prakasha, H.M., Krishnappa, M. and Krishnamurthy, Y.L. "Folk medicine of NR Pura taluk in Chikmagalur district of Karnataka". *Indian Journal of Traditional Knowledge,* Vol. 9, No. 1, 2010, pp. 55-60.

1362. Pramod, C., Sivadasan, M. and Kumar, N. Anil "Ethnobotany of Religious and Supernatural Beliefs of Kurichya of Wayanad district, Kerala, India". *Ethnobotany,* Vol. 15, No. 1-2, 2003, pp. 11-19.

1363. Prasad, L.V. "Indian system of medicine and homeopathy". In Traditional Medicine in Asia, edited by Ranjit Roy Chaudhury and Uton Muchtar Rafei, World Health Organization Regional Office for South-East Asia, New Delhi, 2001, pp. 283-286.

1364. Prasad, R.R. and Kapoor, A.K. "Illness and its cognitive aspect among the Jaad tribals of Central Himalaya". Journal of Social Research, 1982, pp. 1-4.

1365. Prashantkumar, P. and Vidyasagar, G.M. "Documentation of traditional knowledge on medicinal plants of Bidar district, Karnataka". *Indian Journal of Traditional Knowledge,* Vol. 5, No. 3, 2006, pp. 295-299.

1366. Prashantkumar, P. and Vidyasagar, G. M. "Traditional knowledge on medicinal plants used for the treatment of skin diseases in Bidar district, Karnataka". *Indian Journal of Traditional Knowledge,* Vol. 7, No. 2, 2008, pp. 273-276.

1367. Precope, J. "Medicine, magic and mythology", Delhi, Chand and Company Publishers, 1954.

1368. Premila, M. S. "Ayurvedic herbs-A clinical guide to the healing plants of traditional Indian medicine". The Haworth Press, Binghamton, N.Y., 2006, p. 368.

1369. Priyadarshan, S.S. "Herbal veterinary medicines in an ancient Sanskrit work– The Garuda Purana". *Ethnobotany,* Vol. 3, No. 1-2, 1991, pp. 82-87.

1370. Pullaiah, T. "Encyclopaedia of World medicinal plants (in 5 Vols.)". New Delhi, Regency Publications, 2006.

1371. Pullaiah, T. "Medicinal plants in India (in 2 Vols.)". New Delhi, Regency Publication, 2002, p. 580.

1372. Pullaiah, T. and Dharmachandra Kumar "Herbal plants in Mannanur forest, Mahaboobnagar district, Andhra Pradesh". In Ethnobotany and medicinal plants of Indian Sub-continent, edited by J. K. Maheshwari, Jodhpur, India Scientific Publishers, 2000.

1373. Punjani, Bhasker L. "Ethnomedicinal Uses of Vitaceae

among the Tribals of North Gujarat". *Ethnobotany,* Vol. 16, No. 1-2, 2004, pp. 83-85.

1374. Punjani, Bhasker L. "Ethno-Medicobotanical Study of Kathodi Tribe of Sabarkantha in Gujarat". *Ethnobotany,* Vol. 18, No. 1-2, 2006, pp. 135-138.

1375. Punjani, Bhasker L. "Herbal folk medicines used for urinary complaints in tribals pockets of northeast Gujarat". *Indian Journal of Traditional Knowledge,* Vol. 9, No. 1, 2010, pp. 126-130.

1376. Punjani, Bhasker L. "Plants used in Contact Therapy by Tribals of Sabarkantha: (Gujarat)". *Ethnobotany,* Vol. 14, No. 1-2, 2002, pp. 57-59.

1377. Puri H. S. and Pandey, G. "Glimpses into the crude drugs of Sikkim". Bulletin of Medico-Ethno-Botanical Research, Vol. 1, 1980, pp. 55-71.

1378. Puri, H.S. "Traditional herbal medicines for modern times, Vol. 2, Rasayana: Ayurvedic herbs for longevity and rejuvenation". Journal of Alternative and Complementary Medicine, Vol. 9, No. 2, 2003, pp. 331-332.

1379. Purkayasha, Jubilee and Nath, Subhan C. "Biological activities of ethnomedicinal claims of some plant species of Assam". *Indian Journal of Traditional Knowledge,* Vol. 5, No. 2, 2006, pp. 229-236.

1380. Purkayastha, Jubilee, Dutta, Malakshmi and Nath, Subhan C. "Ethnomedicinal plants from Dibru-saikhowa biosphere reserve, Assam". *Indian Journal of Traditional Knowledge,* Vol. 6, No. 3, 2007, pp. 477-480.

1381. Purohit, A.N. "Himalayan medicinal plants– Focus on Uttarakhand". In Himalayan Biodiversity: Action Plan, Gyanodaya Prakashan, Nainital, 1997, pp. 91-110.

1382. Purohit, V.P., Silas, R.A. and Gaur, R.D. "Ethnobotanical studies of some medicinal plants used in skin diseases from Raath (Pauri) Garhwal Himalaya". Journal of Science Research Plant Medicine, Vol. 6, 1986, pp. 39-47.

1383. Purohit, V. P., Silas, R. A. and Gaur, R. D. "Vaidyas and herbal remedies in North Bengal: some useful data about plant use". Folklore, Vol. 27, No. 8, 1986, pp. 155-161.

1384. Pushpalata, H., Sauthan, T.R., Pattanshetty, J.K. and

Holla, B.V. "Folk medicines from some rural areas of Bangalore district". Aryavaidyan, Vol. 12, No. 3/4, 1990, pp. 215-219.

1385. Pushpangadan, P. "Amrithapala (Janakia arayalpatra, Joseph and Chandrasekharan): A new drug from the Kani tribe of Kerala". Ancient Science Life, Vol. 9. No. 4, April 1990, pp. 215-219.

1386. Rabish Chandra and others "Ethnomedicinal formulations used by traditional herbal practitioners of Ranchi, Jharkhand". *Indian Journal of Traditional Knowledge,* Vol. 6, No. 4, 2007, pp. 599-601.

1387. Radhakrishnan, V. N. "The Traditional Medicine of Kanikkars". Kalpadhenu, Vol. 13, No. 3, 1985.

1388. Ragupathy, S. and Mahadevan, A. "Traditional medicine and ethno-botany among Dravidian tribal communities". In Encyclopaedia of Dravidian tribes, edited by T. M. Menon, Thiruvananthapuram, International School of Dravidian Linguistic, 1996, pp. 1-5.

1389. Ragupathy, Subramanyam and Newmaster, Steven G. "Valorizing the 'Irulas' traditional knowledge of medicinal plants in the Kodiakkarai Reserve Forest, India". Journal of Ethnobiology and Ethnomedicine, Vol. 5, No. 10, 2009. (http://www. ethnobiomed. com/content/5/1/10)

1390. Ragupathy, Subramanyam and others "Consensus of the 'Malasars' traditional aboriginal knowledge of medicinal plants in the Velliangiri holy hills, India". Journal of Ethnobiology and Ethnomedicine Vol. 4, No. 8, 2008.

1391. Rai, Arun K., Palni, Uma and Tamang, Jyoti Prakash "Traditional knowledge of the Himalayan people on production of indigenous meat products". *Indian Journal of Traditional Knowledge,* Vol. 8, No. 1, 2009, pp. 104-109.

1392. Rai, B.K. and Rai, Arvinder "Use of Fungas in Folk Medicine: for family planning among Baiga tribe". Folklore, Vol. 33, No. 3, 1992, p. 65.

1393. Rai, Brajesh Kumar, Ayachi, Shivshanker and Rai, Arvinder "A note on ethno-myco-medicines from central India". In Ethnobotany and medicinal Plants of Indian Sub-continent, edited by J. K. Maheshwari, Jodhpur, India Scientific Publishers, 2000.

1394. Rai, M. K. "Plants use as medicine by the tribals of Chhindwara district (M.P.)". Journal of Economic and Taxonomic Botany, Vol. 7, 1985, pp. 385-387.

1395. Rai, M.K. and Shukla, H.D. "A critical study on plants of Ramacharitmanas: A religous Book of Hindus". SEBS Newsletter, Vol. 8, 1989, pp. 3-4.

1396. Rai, M.K., Pandey, A.K. and Acharya, D. "Ethno-medicinal plants used by Gond tribe of Bhanadehi, district Chhindwara, Madhya Pradesh". Journal of Non-timber Forest Products, Vol. 7, No. 3/4, 2000, pp. 237-241.

1397. Rai, Rajiva Kumar and Dixit, S.K. "Ancient traditional technology for preparing bhasmas of metals and minerals with special reference to preparation of tamra bhasma". *Indian Journal of Traditional Knowledge,* Vol. 2, No. 1, 2003, pp. 15-21.

1398. Rai, S.C. "Apatani paddy-cum-fish cultivation: An indigenous hill farming system of North East India". *Indian Journal of Traditional Knowledge,* Vol. 4, No. 1, 2005, pp. 65-71.

1399. Raj Pramukh, K.E. and Palkumar, P.D.S. "Indigenous Knowledge: Implications in Tribal Health and Disease". Studies of Tribes and Tribals, Vol. 4, No. 1, 2006, pp. 1-6.

1400. Raj, K.P.S. and Parmar, R.M. "Garlic-condiments and medicine". Indian drugs, Vol. 15, 1978, pp. 205-210.

1401. Rajadurai, M., Vidhya, V. G. and Ramya, M. "Ethno-medicinal plants used by the traditional healers of Pachamalai hills, Tamil Nadu, India". Studies on Ethno-medicine, Vol. 3, No. 1, 2009, pp. 39-41.

1402. Rajagopalan, C.R. "Indigenous knowledge/CFS (Centre Folk Studies) experience". *Indian Journal of Traditional Knowledge,* Vol. 2, No. 4, 2003.

1403. Rajakumar, N. and Shivanna, M. B. "Traditional veterinary healthcare practices in Shimoga district of Karnataka, India". *Indian Journal of Traditional Knowledge,* Vol. 11, No. 2, 2012, pp. 283-287.

1404. Rajakumar, N. and Shivanna, M. B. "Traditional Herbal Medicinal Knowledge in Sagar Taluk of Shimoga District, Karnataka, India". Indian Journal of Natural Products and resources, Vol. 1, No. 1, 2010, pp. 102-108.

1405. Rajan, S. and Sethuraman, M. "Trditional veterinary practices in rural areas of Dindigul district, Tamil Nadu, India". Indigenous Knowwledge and development Monitor, Vol. 5, No. 3, 1997.

1406. Rajan, S., Jayendran, M., Sethuraman, M. "Medico-ethnobotany: A study on the Kattunayaka tribe of Nilgiri hills, Tamil Nadu". Journal of Natural Remedies, Vol. 3, 2002, pp. 68-72.

1407. Rajan, S., Sethuraman, M., Manikandan, P. L. Arul and Jayendran, M. "Folk herbal therapeutics of six Nilgiri tribes: Resources for Scientific Research and Development". In Traditional Knowledge in Contemporary Societies: Challenges and Apportunities, edited by Kamal K. Misra and K. K. Basa, IGRMS, Bhopal and Pratibha Prakashan, Delhi, 2007, pp. 250-257.

1408. Rajendran, A. and Henry, A. N. "Plants used by the tribe Kadar in Anamalai Hills of Tamil Nadu". *Ethnobotany,* Vol. 6, No. 1-2, 1994, pp. 19-24.

1409. Rajendran, A. and Henry, A. N. "Women's indigenous knowledge of gynaecological theraphy and plants". Vanyajati, Vol. 45, No. 1, 1997, pp. 11-14.

1410. Rajendran, A. and Manian, S. "Herbal remedies for diabetes from the Kolli hills, Eastern Ghats, India". Indian Journal of Natural Products and Resources, Vol. 2, No. 3, 2011, pp. 383-386.

1411. Rajendran, A., Rao, N. Rama & Henry, A.N. "Hepatic stimulant plants of Andhra Pradesh, India". In Ethnobotany and medicinal Plants of Indian Sub-continent, edited by J.K. Maheshwari, Jodhpur, India Scientific Publishers, 2000.

1412. Rajendran, A., Rao, N. Rama and Henery, A.N. "Rare and noteworthy plants of the Eastern Ghats in Andhra Pradesh with their Ethnic Uses". *Ethnobotany,* Vol. 9, No. 1-2, 1997, pp. 39-43.

1413. Rajendran, K., Balaji, P. and Basu, M. Jothi "Medicinal plants and their utilization by villagers in southern districts of Tamil Nadu". *Indian Journal of Traditional Knowledge,* Vol. 5, No. 3, 2006, pp. 417-420.

1414. Rajendran, S.M. and Agarwal, S.C. "Medicinal plants

conservation through sacred forests by ethnic tribals of Virudhunagar district, Tamil Nadu". *Indian Journal of Traditional Knowledge,* Vol. 6, No. 2, 2007, pp. 328-333.

1415. Rajendran, S.M., Sekar, K. Chandra and Sundaresan, V. "Ethnomedicinal lore of valaya tribal in seithur hills of Virudunagar district, Tamil Nadu, India". *Indian Journal of Traditional Knowledge,* Vol. 1, No. 1, 2002 pp. 59-71.

1416. Rajith, N. P., Navas, A. and Thaha, A. Muhammad "A study on traditional mother care plants of rural communities of South Kerala". *Indian Journal of Traditional Knowledge,* Vol. 9, No. 1, 2010, pp. 203-208.

1417. Raju, B. Rama "Telugu Folk Medicine: exposition of a folklorologist". Folklore, Vol. 25, No. 8, 1984, pp. 145-155.

1418. Raju, M. Panduranga, Prasanthi, S. and Seetharami, T. V. V. "Tribal Artefacts of Kerala". *Ethnobotany,* Vol. 12, No. 1-2, 2000, pp. 67-71.

1419. Raju, M. Panduranga, Prashant, S., Sheetharami, T. V. V. Reddi "Medicinal plants in folk medicine for women's diseases in use by Konda Reddis". *Indian Journal of Traditional Knowledge,* Vol. 10, No. 3, 2011, pp. 563-567.

1420. Raju, Vatsavaya S. and Reddy, K.N. "Ethnomedicine for dysentery and diarrhoea from Khammam district of Andhra Pradesh". *Indian Journal of Traditional Knowledge,* Vol. 4, No. 4, 2005, pp. 443-447.

1421. Rajwar, G.S. "Exploitation of medicinal plants of Garhwal Himalaya". Science and Environment, Vol. 2, 1984, pp. 37-41.

1422. Rajwar, G.S. "Low altitude medicinal plants of South Garhwal". Bulletin Medico-ethnobotany Research, Vol. 4, 1983, pp. 14-28.

1423. Ram, A. Jeevan, Raja, K. and Reddy, K. Eswara "Medicinal Plant Lore of Sugalis of Gooty Forests, Andhra Pradesh". *Ethnobotany,* Vol. 14, No. 1-2, 2002, pp. 37-42.

1424. Rama Rao, V.V. "Impact of supplementary feeding on tribal pre school children of Andhra Pradesh: An Anthropometric assessment". *Man in India,* Vol. 64, No. 2, 1984, pp. 167-174.

1425. Ramakrishnan, P. S. "Man and Nature: Indigenous wisdom". Humanscape Vol. 8, pp. 5-10.

1426. Ramana Rao, V. V. "Traditional medicines of Chenchus". Tribal Research Institute, Hyderabad, 1982.

1427. Ramesh, A. and B. Hyma "Traditional Indian medicine in practice in an Indian metropolitan city". Social Science and Medicine, Vol. 15D, 1981, pp. 69-81.

1428. Ramunny, Murkot, "Anthropology of Tribal Health and Medicine in Forest Environment-administrators experiences". Paper presented at the National workshop on Anthropology of tribal health and medicine in forest environment Department of KIRTADS, Kozhikode, Kerala, 1987.

1429. Rana, Man and Samant, S.S. "Diversity, indigenous uses and conservation status of medicinal plants in Manali wildlife sanctuary, North western Himalaya". *Indian Journal of Traditional Knowledge,* Vol. 10, No. 3, 2011, pp. 439- 459.

1430. Ranchan, Som P. "Aurotherapy: An Alternate Therapy System". Delhi, Indian Publishers Distributions, 2001, p. 313.

1431. Rani, Geetha "Medicinal plants viz a viz indigenous knowledge among the tribals of Pachamalai hills". *Indian Journal of Traditional Knowledge,* Vol. 9, No. 1, 2010, pp. 209-215.

1432. Ranjan, Priya "A contribution to some of the medicinal plants of Indo-Nepal border area adjointing the districts of Madhubani and Sitamarchi". In Ethnobotany and medicinal plant of Indian subcontinent, edited by J. K. Maheshwari, Saujanya Books, Jodhpur, 2003, p. 672.

1433. Rao, B.T., Lakshmi, B.B., Rao, L.M. "Medico-ethnology and conservation of medicinal plants of Pederu forest division-Visakhapatnam". Ecolology Environment and Conservation, Vol. 7, 2001, pp. 117-131.

1434. Rao, D. Muralidhar and Pullaiah, T. "Ethno-medico-botanical studies in Guntur district of Andhra Pradesh, India". *Ethnobotany,* Vol. 13, No. 1-2, 2001, pp. 40-44.

1435. Rao, K.P. and Sreenamulu, S.H. "Ethnobotany of selected medicinal plants of Srikakulam district, Andhra Pradesh". Ancient Science of Life, Vol. 4, 1985, pp. 238-244.

1436. Rao, M.K.V. and Shanpru, R. "Some plants in the life of Garos of Meghalaya". In Glimpses of Indian Ethnobotany edited by S.K. Jain, New Delhi, Oxford & IBH, 1981, pp. 153-160.

1437. Rao, M.S.A. "Supernatural possession in Kerala". *Man in India,* Vol. 66, No.1, 1986.

1438. Rao, M. V. Krishna and Prasad, O. S. V. D. "Ethno medicines of tribes of Andhra Pradesh". *Man and Life,* Vol. 21, No. 1-2, 1995, pp. 1-18.

1439. Rao, N. Goutham, Reddy, S. Prakash & Vijaya, N. "Indian Medicines in Rural areas of Telangana: some suggestions to Policy and Planning body". *Folklore*, Vol. 29, No. 1, July, pp. 10-13.

1440. Rao, N. S. Balaji, Rajasekhar, D. and Raju, D. Chengal "Ethno-medicinal notes on some plants of Tirumala Hills for Dental Disorders". *Ethnobotany,* Vol. 8, No. 1-2, 1996, pp. 88-91.

1441. Rao, P. Durga, Babu, M. Sudhakar and Rao, V.L. Narasimha "Persistent traditional practices among the tribals of north coastal Andhra Pradesh". *Studies of Tribes and Tribals,* Vol. 4, No. 1, 2006, pp. 53-56.

1442. Rao, R. R. "Ethnobiology in the study and conservation of fragile ecosystems: some issues from the Himalayan region". *Ethnobotany,* Vol. 2, No. 1-2, 1990, pp. 45-55.

1443. Rao, R. R. "Ethnobotanical studies on the flora of Meghalaya-some intersting reports of harbal medicines". In Glimpses of Indian *Ethnobotany,* edited by S. K. Jain, New Delhi, Oxford and IBH, 1981, pp. 137-148.

1444. Rao, R. R. "Ethnobotany of Meghalaya: Medicinal plants used by Khasi and Garo tribes". *Economic Botany*, Vol. 35, No. 1, 1981, pp. 4-9.

1445. Rao, R.R. "Indigenous people and forests: Perspectives of an ethnobotanical study from Nagaland, North East India". In Ethnobiology in Human Welfare edited by S.K. Jain, Deep & Deep Publications, New Delhi, pp. 367-371, 1996.

1446. Rao, R.R. and Hajra, R.K. "Methods of research in ethnobotany". In A Manual of Ethnobotany edied by S.K. Jain, Scientific Publisher, Jodhpur. pp. 33-41, 1987.

1447. Rao, R.R. and Jamir, N.S. "Ethnobotanical Studies in Nagaland-II: 54 medicinal plants used by Nagas". *Journal of Economic and Taxonomic Botany*, Vol. 3, 1982, pp. 11-17.

1448. Rao, V.L.N. and others "Ethnomedicinal practices among Khonds of Visakhapatnam district, Andhra Pradesh". *Indian Journal of Traditional Knowledge,* Vol. 5, No. 2, 2006, pp. 217-219.

1449. Rao, Y.K. "Tribal people and cultivation and collection of medicinal plants from minor and major forest areas". *Nagarjun*, Vol. 21, No. 7, 1978, pp. 34-50.

1450. Rasiya, Beegam A. and Nayar, T. S. "Plants used for natal healthcare in folk medicine of Kerala, India". *Indian Journal of Traditional Knowledge,* Vol. 10, No. 3, 2011, pp. 523-527.

1451. Rasmussen, Susan J. "Only women know trees: medicine women & role of herbal healing in Tuareg culture". *Journal of Anthropology Research*, Vol. 54, No. 2, 1998, 147-171.

1452. Rastogi, Ram P. and Mehrotra, B. N. (eds.) "Compendium of Indian medicinal plants (in 2 Vols.)". Lucknow, Central Drug Research Institute, 1990, p. 1330.

1453. Rath, Swetansu Sekhar "Indian tribes and their urgent and emerging health status: An overview". In Tribal health and medicines, edited by A.K. Kalla and P.C. Joshi, New Delhi: Concept Publishing Co.2004, pp. 46-69.

1454. Rathakrishnan, T., Anandaraja, N. and Ramasubramanian M. "Traditional products and practices of indigenous people inhabiting Ramanathapuram district of Tamil Nadu". *Indian Journal of Traditional Knowledge,* Vol. 7, No. 1, 2008, pp. 23-26.

1455. Rathi, B.S., Baheti, A.M. and Khandelwal, K.R. "Diuretic activity of coconut husk mashi-an ayurvedic formulation". *Indian Journal of Traditional Knowledge,* Vol. 5, No. 4, 2006, pp. 471-473.

1456. Rati, R.N. "Ethno-medicinal practices and sustainable development, Senstive Issues of economic transformation in Chhattisgarh". *Journal of Indian Anthropological Society*, Vol. 40, No. 1, 2005, pp. 65-74.

1457. Ratnam, Venkata and Raju, R.R. Venkata "Folk medicine used for common women ailments by Adivasi in the eastern Ghats of Andhra Pradesh". *Indian Journal of Traditional Knowledge,* Vol. 4, No. 3, 2005, pp. 267-270.

1458. Raut, Ashwini Kumar A. and others "Bhallatak (Semecarpus anacardium Linn.): A review". *Indian Journal of Traditional Knowledge,* Vol. 6, No. 4, 2007, pp. 653-659.

1459. Rawat, G.S. and Pangety, Y.P.S. "A contribution to the ethnobotany of Alpine regions of Kumaun". *Journal of Economic and Taxonomic Botany*, Vol. 11, 1987, pp. 139-148.

1460. Rawat, G.S. and Purohit, A.N. "The need for Alpine Gardens to conserve and multiply rare medicinal herbs ain the Central Himalaya". In Indigenous medicinal plants: including microbes and fungi edited by Purshotam Kaushik, Today and tomorrow's printers and Publishers, New Delhi, 1988, pp. 179-186.

1461. Rawat, G.S., Kalakoti, B.S. & Pangtey, Y.P.S. "Himalaya ki ujharti durlabh sampada". Pahar, 1986, pp. 86-89. [Hindi]

1462. Ray, Aniruddha (ed.) "Tipu Sultan and his age: a collection of seminar papers". Kolkata, Asiatic Society, 2002, p. 204.

1463. Ray, G.S., Chattopadhyay, G. & Biswas, S. "A magico-religious ceremony in connection with the disease of 'Ho Boy'". *Man in India,* Vol. 34, 1954, pp. 194-204.

1464. Ray, J. K. "Alcoholoic beverages in tribal India and their nutritional role". *Man in India,* Vol. 58, No. 4, 1978, pp. 298-326.

1465. Ray, J. K. "Nutritional implications of some cultural practices: Studies in tribal areas of Orissa". In Health and human behaviour edited by B. S. Reddy, Calcutta, All India Institute of hygiene and public health, 1954.

1466. Ray, J.K., Bhattacharya, K.K. & Biswas, S.K. "Diet and nutritional anthropometry of Santals of Purulia". *Bulletin of the Anthropological Survey of India*, Vol. 31, No. 1-2, pp. 1983, 45-70.

1467. Ray, S. N. "Some trees and herbs in rituals and folklore (Bengal and Orissa)". Journal of Anthropological Sociology Bombay, Vol. 14, 1931, pp. 588-604.

1468. Reagan, A. "Plants used by the Hoh and Quilents Indian". *Transactions of the Kansas Academy of Science*, Vol. 37, 1974.

1469. Reddy, A. P. "Genetic relationship between the Chenchu, Irula and yanadi: A reassessment". *Journal of Indian Anthropological Society*, Vol. 18, No.1, 1983, pp. 31-34.

1470. Reddy, K. N., Trimurthulu, G. and Reddy, C. Sudhakar "Plants used by the ethnic people of Krishna district, Andhra Pradesh". *Indian Journal of Traditional Knowledge,* Vol. 9, No. 2, 2010, pp. 313-317.

1471. Reddy, M. Hemambara, Reddy, R.V. and Raju, R.R. Venkata "Rutaceous plants from tribal medicine of Andhra Pradesh". *Ancient Science of Life*, Vol. 17, No. 4, 1998, pp. 251-252.

1472. Reddy, M. Hemambara, Vijayalakshmi, K. & Raju, R. R. Venkata "Native phyto-therapy for snake bite in Nallamalais, Eastern Ghats, India". In Ethnobotany and medicinal plants of Indian Sub-continent, edited by J. K. Maheshwari, Jodhpur, India Scientific Publishers, 2000.

1473. Reddy, P. Ramachandra, Rao, P. Padma and Prabhakar, M. "Ethnomedicinal practices amongst Chenchus of Nagarjunasagar Srisailam Tiger Reserve (NSTR), Andhra Pradesh: plant remedies for cuts, wounds and boils". *Ethnobotany,* Vol. 15, No. 1-2, 2003, pp. 45-55.

1474. Reddy, R.V., Lakshmi, N.V.N. and Raju, R.R. Venkata "Ethnomedicine for Ephemeral Fevers and Anthrax in Cattle from the Hills of Cuddapah district, Andhra Pradesh, India". *Ethnobotany,* Vol. 9, No. 1-2, 1997, pp. 94-96.

1475. Reddy, S. Krishna "Folk Medicine among the Yerukula's: an anthropological study". *Folklore*, Vol. 32, No. 4, 1991, pp. 62-66.

1476. Rethy, P., Singh, B. and Kagyung, R. "Ethnobotanical studies of dehang- debang biosphere reserve of Arunachal Pradesh with special reference to Memba tribe". *Indian Journal of Traditional Knowledge,* Vol. 9, No. 1, 2010, pp. 61-67.

1477. Revathi, P. and Parimelazhagan, T. "Traditional knowledge on medicinal plants used by the Irula tribe Hasanur

Hills,Erode district, Tamil Nadu, India". *Ethnobotanical Leaflets*, Vol. 14, 2010, pp. 136-60.

1478. Reyner, J. H. "Poisoned medicine: the study and treatment of the causative factors in illness". New York, Samuel Weiser, 1974, p. 139.

1479. Ringmichon, C. L., Shimpi, Shraddha and Gopalkrishnan, Bindu "Some noteworthy antipyretic herbal remedies used by Naga tribes in Manipur". *Ethnobotany,* Vol. 23, No. 1&2, 2011, pp. 82-85.

1480. Rivers, W.H.R. "Medicine, magic and religion". New York, Harcourt, Brace, 1924.

1481. Rizvi, S. N. H. "Health practices of the Jaunsaris- A socio-cultural analysis". In Tribal health: Socio-Cultural dimentions, edited by Buddhadeb Chaudhuri, New Delhi, Inter India, 1986, pp. 223-246.

1482. Rohilla, P. P. and Mathur, D. C. "Indigenous traditional knowledge used for animals treatment in Pali". *Indian Farming*, Vol. 53, No. 6, 2003, pp. 17-19.

1483. Rosakutty, P. J., Roslin, S. Stella and Ignacimuthu, S. "Some traditional folklore medicinal plants of Kanyakumari district (Tamil Nadu)". In Ethnobotany and medicinal plant of Indian subcontinent, edited by J. K. Maheshwari, Saujanya Books, Jodhpur, 2003, p. 672.

1484. Ross, Ivan A. "Medicinal plants of the world: chemical constituents, traditional and modern medicinal uses". New Jersey, Humana Press, 2001, p. 487.

1485. Rothe, S.P. "Ethnomedicinal plants from Katepurna wildlife sanctuary of Akola district". *Indian Journal of Traditional Knowledge,* Vol. 2, No. 4, 2003, pp. 378-382.

1486. Rothe, S.P. and Ukesh, C.S. "Ethno-medico-botanical study from Ambabarva wild life sanctuary of Buldhana district". *Vanyajati*, Vol. 59, No. 3, 2011, pp. 35-36.

1487. Rothe, S.P., Pethe, A.S. and Kothale, K.V. "Ethnomedico botanical study from tribal regions of West Vidarbha (M.S.)". *Vanyajati*, Vol. 56, No. 3, 2008, pp. 11-16.

1488. Rout, S. D., Panda, T. and Mishra, N. "Ethno- medicinal plants used to cure different diseases by tribals of Mayurbhanj disctrict of north Orissa". *Studies on Ethno-medicine,* Vo. 3, No. 1, 2009, pp. 27-32.

1489. Rove, Michael R. "Indigenous People and Environmental Politics". *Annual Review of Anthropology*, Vol. 35, 2006, pp. 191-208.

1490. Roy, Babul "Folk perception of disease and curative measures among the zeme Nagas of north cachar hills in Assam". *Journal of Indian Anthropological Society,* Vol. 39, No. 1, 2004, pp. 57-66.

1491. Roy, G. P. and Chaturvedi, K. K. "Ethno-medicinal trees of Abujh-Marh: area, Peser Bastar district in Madhya Pradesh" *Folklore*, Vol. 27, No. 5, 1986, pp. 95-98.

1492. Roy, G. P. and Chaturvedi, K. K. "Ethnomedicinal trees of Abujh-Marh area, Madhya Pradesh". *Folklore*, Vol. 27, 1986, pp. 95-100.

1493. Roy, G.P. and Chaturvedi, K.K. "Folk-lore claims of Sukula Jadi: Heteropogon Contortus (L.) P. Beauv. Ex. Roem and Schult". *Folklore*, Vol. 27, No. 5, 1986, pp. 99-100.

1494. Roy, S. N. "Some popular supersititions of Orissa". *Man in India,* Vol. 5, 1925, pp. 210-234.

1495. Roy, Siddhartha and Das, A.P. "An effective remedy for Jaundice with Thespesia Populnea from Purullia distric of West Bengal (India)". *Ethnobotany,* Vol.16, No.1-2, 2004, pp. 50-51.

1496. Rubel, Arthur J. and Hass, Michael R. "Ethnomedicine". In Handbook of Medical Anthropology: Contemporary Theory and Method edited by Carolyn F. Sargent and Thomas M. Johnson, Westport, CT, Greenwood Press, 1996, pp. 113-150.

1497. Russell, R. V. and Hiralala, R. B. "Tribes and castes of the Central Provinces of India (in 4 Vols.)". New Delhi, Cosmo Publications, 1975.

1498. Sabar, Bhubaneswar "Ethno-veterinary practice among the Chuktia Bhunjia tribe of Nuapada district of Orissa". *Man and Life,* Vol. 36, No. 3-4, 2010, pp. 61-74.

1499. Sachan, Nikhil K. "Sociological aspects in community health and medicine". *Man and Life,* Vol. 33, No. 1-2, 2007, pp. 89-100.

1500. Sachchidananda "Socio-cultural dimensions of tribal health". *Journal of Social and economic studies*, Vol. 3, No. 4, 1986, pp. 89-401.

1501. Sadique, J. (ed.) "Satellite symposium on traditional medicine as adjunct to Asian Congress of pharmacology". Thanjavur, Tamil University, 1986, p. 283.

1502. Sagar, M. P., Ahlawat, O. P. and Raj, Dev "Indigenous technical knowledge about the use of spent mushroom substrate". *Indian Journal of Traditional Knowledge,* Vol. 8, No. 2, 2009, pp. 242-248.

1503. Saha, Kshanika "Indian medical text in Central Asia". Calcutta, Firma KLM Private, 1985, p. 55.

1504. Saha, Mridula "History of Indian medicine based on Vedic literature: Satapatha Brahmana". Calcutta, Asiatic Society, 1999, p. 79.

1505. Saha, N. N. "Vegetable juice therapy: how to get relief from drug addiction and other maladies". Calcutta, Firma KLM Private, 1996. p.118.

1506. Sahai, Suman "Impartance of indigenous knowledge in IPR system". *Economic and Political Weekly,* Vol. 31, No. 47, 1996, pp. 3043-3045.

1507. Sahay, K. N. "Tree cult in tribal culture". *Folklore*, Vol. 5, No. 7, 1964, pp. 7-18.

1508. Sahay, Vijoy S. and Duary, Nabakumar "The fading traditional tribal institutions of Chotanagpur: A study of the Oraons and the Mundas". *Vanyajati*, Vol. 46, No. 4, 1998, pp. 20-28.

1509. Saheb, Yaseen, Prasad, M. Rajendra and Bhanu, B. Ananda "The health profile of the Irula tribe of Tamil Nadu". *South Asian Anthropologist*, Vol. 8, No. 1, 2008, pp. 13-22.

1510. Sahoo, A. K. and Mudgal, V. "Less known Ethnobotanical Uses of Plants of Phulbani district, Orissa, India". *Ethnobotany,* Vol. 7, No. 1-2, 1995, pp. 63-67.

1511. Sahoo, B. B. and Satapathy, K. B. "Plants used by the tribals and rural folks for common ailments in Jaipur district Orissa." *Ethnobotany,* Vol. 21, No. 1-2, 2009, pp. 107-111.

1512. Sahoo, K. N. and others "A life saving medicine made by a vanishing species". *Indian Journal of Traditional Knowledge,* Vol. 4, No. 2, 2005, pp. 132-138.

1513. Sahu, Dinesh Kuma and Mukherjee, B. M. "The Knowledge that helps indigenous people: An anthropological exploration". In Traditional Knowledge in Contemporary Societies: Challenges and Apportunities, edited by Kamal K. Misra and K. K. Basa, IGRMS, Bhopal and Pratibha Prakashan, Delhi, 2007, pp. 146-152.

1514. Sahu, S.C., Dhal, N.K. and Mohanty, R.C. "Potential medicinal plants used by the tribal of Deogarh district, Orissa, India". *Studies on ethno-medicine*, Vol. 4, No. 1, 2010, pp. 53-61.

1515. Sahu, S. K. "Growth of medical anthropology in India: issues and perspectives". Proceedings of XI Conference on Ethnographic and folk culture Society. 1984.

1516. Sahu, S. K. "Health culture of the Oraons in the contex of different health institution". *Ethnomedicine*, Vol. 6, 1980, pp.167-182.

1517. Sahu, S.K. "Role of anthropologists in community health (mimeograph)" 1981.

1518. Sahu, S. K. "Social dimensions of health of tribals in India: A case study of Oraons of Orissa". In Tribal Health: Socio-cultural dimensions, edited by Buddhadeb Chaudhuri, New Delhi, Inter India, 1986, pp. 303-310.

1519. Sahu, S. K. "Social dimentions of human health and disease in India". Proceedings of International Conference on Man and Environment, 1983, Calcutta.

1520. Sahu, T. R. "An ethnobotanical study of Madhya Pradesh I: Plants used against various disorders among tribal women". *Ancient Science of life*, Vol. 1, 1982, pp. 178-181.

1521. Said, Hakim Mohammed "The influence of traditional medicine upon modern medicine". *Impact of Science on Society,* Vol. 36, No. 3, 1986, pp. 307-312.

1522. Saigal, Omesh "The art and science of healing". *Discovery India,* Vol. 13, No. 8, 2000, pp. 6-7.

1523. Saikia, Bipul "Ethno medicinal uses of plognum strigosum mishing tribes of Gopur sub- division in Somnitpur district, Assam". *Ethnobotany,* Vol. 20, No. 1-2, 2008, pp. 150-151.

1524. Saikia, Bipul and Borthakur, S. K. "Use of medicinal plants in animal healthcare- A case study from Gohpur, Assam". *Indian Journal of Traditional Knowledge,* Vol. 9, No. 1, 2010, pp. 49-51.

1525. Saikia, Padma Dhar "Studies in Dafla social and religious life". Department of Tribal Culture and Folklore Research, Assam, 1964, p. 70.

1526. Saini, D.C. "Ethnobotany of Tharus of Basti district, Uttar Pradesh". In Ethnobotany and medicinal plants of Indian Sub-continent, edited by J. K. Maheshwari, Jodhpur, India Scientific Publishers, 2000.

1527. Saiprasad Goud, P. and Pullaiah, T. "Ethnobotany of Kurnool district- some wild plants used as food". In Ethnobotany and medicinal plants of Indian Sub-continent, edited by J. K. Maheshwari, Jodhpur, India Scientific Publishers, 2000.

1528. Sajem Albert L., Gosai, Kuldip "Traditional use of medicinal plants by the Jaintia Tribes in North Cachar Hills district of Assam, northeast India". *Journal of Ethnobiology and Ethnomedicine*, Vol. 2, No. 33, 2006. (Bio Med Central Full Text)

1529. Sajem, Albert L. and Gosai, Kuldip "Ethnobotanical investigations among the Lushai tribes in North Cachar hills district of Assam, Northeast India". *Indian Journal of Traditional Knowledge,* Vol. 9, No. 1, 2010, pp. 108-113.

1530. Sakarkar, D. M., Sakarkar, U. M. and Jaiswal, S. B. "Essence of ayurveda: The traditional medical science". *Indian Journal of Traditional Knowledge,* Vol. 2, No. 4, 2003, pp. 333-345.

1531. Sakhuja, Swarna Lata "The medical and health care of women: Sociological Study of rural and tribal Hilly areas in Uttaranchal Pradesh". New Delhi, Gyan Publishing House, 2008, p. 220.

1532. Saklani, Bina "Mechanical strategies in folk medicine in Rawain (Garhwal Himalaya)". *Indian Anthropoogist*, Vol. 22, No. 2, 1992, pp. 31-40.

1533. Saklani, Bina "Mechanical strategies in folk medicine in Rawain". *Indian Anthropoogist*, Vol. 25 No. 2, 1995, pp. 25-33.

1534. Saklani, Pradeep Mohan "Traditional practice and knowledge of wild plants among the ethnic communities of Garhwal Himalaya". *Puratattva*, Vol. 29, 1998, pp. 89-99.

1535. Salam, S., Jamir, N. S. and Singh, P. K. "Ethnomedicinal studies on Tangkhul-Naga tribe in Ukhrul district, Manipur". *Ethnobotany,* Vol. 23, No. 1-2, 2011, pp. 129-134.

1536. Samal, Prasanna K. and Dhyani, Pitamber P. "Gender in the management of indigenous knowledge: Reflections from Indian Central Himalaya". *Current Science,* Vol. 91, No. 1, 2006, pp. 104-108.

1537. Samal, Prasanna K., Dhyani, Pitamber P. and Dollo, Mihin "Indigenous medicinal practices of Bhotia tribal community in Indian central Himalaya". *Indian Journal of Traditional Knowledge,* Vol. 9, No. 1, 2010, pp. 140-144.

1538. Samal, Prasanna K., Shah, Anubha and Tiwari, Sushil "Indigenous animal health care practices in Indian central Himalaya: Empirical evidences". *Indian Journal of Traditional Knowledge,* Vol. 2, No. 1, 2003, pp. 40-50.

1539. Samal, Prasanna K., Shah, Anubha and Tiwari, Sushil C. "Indigenous healthcare practices and their linkages with bioresource conservation and socio-economic development". *Indian Journal of Traditional Knowledge,* Vol. 3, No. 1, 2004, pp. 12-26.

1540. Samant, S.S. "Himalaya ki jari bootiya". In Jav Vivvdhata Sanrakshan Mai Janta Ki Bhagidhari (Jav Vividhata Sanrakshan Vibhag), GBPIHED Kosi-Katarmal, Almora, 1995, pp. 32-47. [Hindi]

1541 Samant, S.S. and Mehta, I.S. "The folklore medicinal plants of Johar Valley Higher Pants of Indian Subcontinent". *Additional Series of Indian Journal of Forestry,* Vol. 3, 1994, pp. 143-159.

1542. Samant, S. S. and Pangety, Y. P. S. "Diversity of Ichthyotoxic plants of Kumaun Himalaya". *Indian Journal Forestry,* Vol. 18, No. 1, 1995, pp. 80-86.

1543. Samant, S.S., Dhar, U. & Palni, L.M.S. "Medicinal plants of Indian Himalaya: Diversity, Distribution Potential Value". Himavikas Publication No. 13. Gyanodaya Prakashan, Nainital, 1998.

1544. Samant, S.S., Dhar, U. & Rawal, R.S. "Diversity, distribution and indigenous uses of threatened medicinal plants of Askot wildlife sanctuary in west Himalaya:

conservation and management perspectives". In Himalayan medicinal plants: potential and prospects edited by S. S. Samant, U. Dhar and L. M. S. Palni, Gyanodaya Prakasan, Nainital, pp. 167-185, 2001.

1545. Samati, H. "Kitchen garden plants of Pnar Tribe in Jaintia Hills district, Meghalaya". *Ethnobotany,* Vol. 16, No. 1-2, 2004, pp. 125-130.

1546. Samuel, J. Jarunyal and Andrews, B. "Traditional medicinal plants wealth of Pachalur and Periyur Hamlets Dindigul district, Tamil Nadu". *Indian Journal of Traditional Knowledge,* Vol. 9, No. 2, 2010, pp. 264-270.

1547. Samvatsar, S. and Diwanji, V. B. "Plant sources for the treatment of jaundice in the tribals of wesern Madhya Pradesh of India". *Journal of Ethnopharmacology,* Vol. 73, 2000, pp. 313-316.

1548. Samvatsar, Swati "Plants used for the treatment of different types of fevers by Bhils and its subtribes in India". *Indian Journal of Traditional Knowledge,* Vol. 3, No. 1, 2004, pp. 96-100.

1549. Samwatsar, Swati and Diwanji, V. B. "House and household of tribals of western M.P.: an ethnobotanical study". In Ethnobotany and medicinal plants of Indian Sub-continent, edited by J. K. Maheshwari, Jodhpur, India Scientific Publishers, 2000.

1550. Samwatsar, Swati and Diwanji, V.B. "Plants used for skin diseases, cuts, wounds and bruises by the tribals of western M.P.". In Ethnobotany and medicinal plants of Indian sub-continent, edited by J.K. Maheshwari, Jodhpur, India Scientific Publishers, 2000.

1551. Samwatsar, Swati, and Diwanji, V.B. "Plants used in snake, scorpion and insect bites/stings by Adibasis of Jhabua (M.P.) India". In Ethnobotany and medicinal plants of Indian sub-continent, edited by J. K. Maheshwari, Jodhpur, India Scientific Publishers, 2000.

1552. Sandhya, B., Thomas, S., Isabel, W. and Shenbagarathai, R. "Ethnomedicinal plants used by the Valaiyan community of Piranmalai hills (Reserved forest), Tamil Nadu, India – A pilot study". *African journal of Traditional, Complementary and Alternative Medicines,* Vol. 3, No. 1, 2006, pp. 101-114.

1553. Sanilkumar, M.G. and Thomas, K. John "Indigenous medicinal usages of some macrophytes of the Muriyad wetland in Vembanad-Kol, Ramsar site, Kerala". *Indian Journal of Traditional Knowledge,* Vol. 6, No. 2, 2007 pp. 365-367.

1554. Sankara Narayanan, A. S. and Sashiraj, Narmatha "Socio-cultural and ethno-botanical studies (on Irula tribe) of Sholayur Panchayat in Attappady, Kerala". *Man and Life,* Vol. 13, No. 3-4, 1987, pp. 181-200.

1555. Sapu, Changkija and Yogendra Kumar "Ethnobotanicl folk practices and beliefs of the Ao-Nagas in Nagaland, India". *Ethnobotany,* Vol. 8, No. 1-2, 1996, pp. 26-30.

1556. Sarangi, N. and Sahu, R. K. "Ethno-medicinal plant used in venereal and gynaecological disorders in Kalahandi, Orissa". *Ethnobotany,* Vol. 16, No. 1-2, 2004, pp. 16-20.

1557. Saraswathy, Ariamuthu, Suganthan, Joy and Vijayalakshmi, R. "Evaluation of an ayurvedic compound formulation-agnimukha curna". *Indian Journal of Traditional Knowledge,* Vol. 6, No. 2, 2007, pp. 298-306.

1558. Saraswati, Baidyanath "Tribal Ayurveda must we destroy It". Paper presented at the National Workshop on Tribal Health and Medicine in Forest Environment, Department of KIRTADS, Kozhikode, Kerala, 1987.

1559. Sardana, Virender "Indigenous technical knowledge of farmers since ancient time". *Indian Farming,* Vol. 51, No. 8, 2001, pp. 13-14.

1560. Sarin, Y.K. "Some less-known but effective Folk Remedies in North-West Himalayan Region". *Ethnobotany,* Vol. 2, No. 1-2, 1990, pp. 39-43.

1561. Sarkar, Amitabha and Dasgupta, Samira "Perception of indigenous knowledge for health care among Bastar tribes". *The Eastern Anthropologist,* Vol. 59, No. 3-4, 2006, pp. 453-455.

1562. Sarkar, Amitabha and Dixit, Vinod Kumar "Use of herbal medicine in tribal Bastar". *Man and Life,* Vol. 25, No. 3-4, 1999, pp. 197-208.

1563. Sarkar, B. N. "Pàlāmar C - Line polymorphism among the Negrito tribes of Andaman Island". *South Asian Anthropologist,* Vol. 11, No. 2, 1990, pp. 49-54.

1564. Sarkar, Eisha "Tribal medicine in the 21st century". (http://www.timeswellness.com/article/6/20091214200912111853472952 8a81b1/Tribal-medicine-in-the-21st-century.html)

1565. Sarkar, R. M. "Dimensions of folk medicine traditions in human society with special reference to rural Bengal". *Man in India,* Vol. 73, No. 4, 1993, pp. 327-341.

1566. Sarker, Profulla C. "Ethno-religiosity and practice of initiation rites in rural Bangladesh: A qualitative analysis". *Man in India,* Vol. 68, No. 1, 1988, pp. 84-92.

1567. Sarma, Chandana and Medhi, Birinchi K. "Beliefs integral to ethno-medicinal plants in a rural context of Assam". In Intangible Cultural Heritage of Assam, edited by Kishor. K. Basa and Brinchi K. Medhi, IGRMS, Bhopal & Pratibha Prakashan, Delhi, 2008, pp. 271-282.

1568. Sarma, S.K., Bhattacharjya, D.K. and Devi, B. "Traditional use of herbal medicines by Madahi Tribe of Nalbari district of Assam". *Ethnobotany,* Vol. 14, No. 1-2, 2002, pp. 103-111.

1569. Sarma, S. K., Bhattacharya, D. K. and Devi, B. "Medicinal plants used by Bodo tribe of Nalbari district in Assam". *Ethnobotany,* Vol. 13, No. 1-2, 2001, pp. 135-139.

1570. Sarmah, P. V. "Bhava Misra-a land mark in the history of Indian medicine". *Journal of Research in Indian Medicine,* Vol. 7, No. 1, 1972, pp. 63-75.

1571. Sarmah, R., Arunachalam, A. and Adhikari, D. "Indigenous technical knowledge and resource utilization of lisus in the south eastern part of Namdapha park, Arunachal". *Indian Journal of Traditional Knowledge,* Vol. 5, No. 1, 2006, pp. 51-56.

1572. Sarman, P. V. "Drugs as land mark of the history of Indian medicine". *Journal of Research in Indian Medicine*, Vol. 8, No.4, 1973, pp. 86-93.

1573. Sasi, R., Rajendran, A. and Aravindhan, V. "Ethno-hair tonic percepts in Velliangiri hills of South Western Ghats". *Ethnobotany,* Vol. 22, No. 1-2, 2010, pp. 107-110.

1574. Satyavati, G.V., Gupta, A.K. and Tandon, N. "Medicinal plants of India, Vol. II". Indian Council of Medical Research, New Delhi, 1987.

1575. Satyavati, G.V., Raina, M.K. and Sharma, M. "Medicinal plants of India, Vol. 1". New Delhi, Indian council of medical research, 1976.

1576. Saunders, Lyle "Healing Ways". In Readings in Anthroplogy edited by J. D. Jennings and E. A. Hoebel, New York, Mc Graw-Hill Book Company, 1954.

1577. Saxena, H. O., Brahman, M. and Dutta, P.K. "Ethnobotanical studies in Orissa". In Glimpses of Indian Ethnobotany, edited by S. K. Jain, New Delhi, Oxford & IBH, 1981, pp. 232-244.

1578. Sayed, M. D. "Traditional medicine in health care". *Journal of Ethnopharmacology,* Vol. 2, 1980, pp. 19-22.

1579. Sayed, Nudrat Z., Deo, Richa and Mukundan, Usha "Herbal remedies used by Warlis of Dahanu to induce lactation in nursing mothers". *Indian Journal of Traditional Knowledge,* Vol. 6, No. 4, 2007, pp. 602-605.

1580. Sayeed-ud-din, M. "Some of the common flowering plants of the Hyderabad state, their distribution, economic and medicinal importance". *Journal of Asiatic Society,* Vol. 1, No. 2, pp. 1935, 9-92.

1581. Scharfe, Hartmut "The doctrine of the three humors in traditional Indian medicine and the alleged antiquity of Tamil Siddha medicine". Journal of the American Oriental Society, Vol. 119, 1999, pp. 609-629.

1582. Schoffeleers, Mathew "Christ as the medicine-man and the medicine-man as Christ". *Man and Life,* Vol. 8, No. 1-2, 1982, pp. 11-28.

1583. Schultes, R. E. "The role of the ethnobotanist in the search for new medicinal plants". *Lloydia*, Vol. 25, 1962, pp. 257-266.

1584. Schultes, Richard Evans "Plants of the gods: origins of hallucinogenic use". London, Hutchinson, 1979, p. 192.

1585. Sebastian, M. K. and Bhandari, M. M. "Magico-Religious Beliefs about Plants: among the Bhills of Udaipur district of Rajasthan". *Folklore*, Vol. 25, No. 4, 1984, pp. 77-79.

1586. Sebastian, M. K. and Bhandari, M. M. "Medicinal plant lore of Udaipur district, Rajasthan". *Bulletin of Medico-ethno-Botanical Research,* Vol. 5, 1984, pp. 122-134.

1587. Seetharam, Y N, Chalageri, Gururaj and Haleshi, C. "Folk Medicine and Ethnomedicine of North-Eastern Karnataka". *Ethnobotany,* Vol. 11, No. 1-2, 1999, pp. 32-37.

1588. Sekar, S and Mariappan, S. "Traditionally fermented biomedicines, arishtas and asavas from ayurveda". *Indian Journal of Traditional Knowledge,* Vol. 7, No. 4, 2008, pp. 548-556.

1589. Sekar, S. "Traditional alcoholic beverages from Ayurveda and their role on human health". *Indian Journal of Traditional Knowledge,* Vol. 6, No. 1, 2007, pp. 144-149.

1590. Sekar, S. and Mariappan, S."Usage of traditional fermented products by Indian rural folks and IPR". *Indian Journal of Traditional Knowledge,* Vol. 6, No. 1, 2007, pp. 111-120.

1591. Selvanayagam, Z. Emmanuel and Gnanavendan, S. G. "Antisnake venom botanicals from ethnomedicine". *Journal of Herbs, Spices and Medicinal Plants*, Vol. 2, No. 4, 1994, pp. 45-100.

1592. Semwal, D. P., Saradhi, P. Pardha and Sajwan, B.S. "Medicinal plants used by local Vaidyas in Ukhimath block, Uttarakhand". *Indian Journal of Traditional Knowledge,* Vol. 9, No. 3, 2010, pp. 480-485.

1593. Sen, Aniruddha and Ghosh, P. D. "A note on the ethnobotanical studies of some pteridophytes in Assam". *Indian Journal of Traditional Knowledge,* Vol. 10, No. 2, 2011, pp. 292-295.

1594. Sen, S. K. and Behera, L. M. "Ethnomedicinal Plants used against Skin Diseases in Bargarh district in Orissa". *Ethnobotany,* Vol. 15, No. 1-2, 2003, pp. 90-96.

1595. Sen, S. K. and Behera, L. M. "Traditional use of herbal medicines against headache and migraine by the tribals of Bargarh district of Orissa". *Ethnobotany,* Vol. 21, No.1-2, 2009, pp. 127-130.

1596. Sen, S.K., Panda, H.S. and Behera, L.M. "Cordia Macleodii (Ehretiaceae): a wounderful wound healer from Bargarh district, Orissa". *Ethnobotany,* Vol.17, No.1-2, 2005, pp. 191-192.

1597. Sen, Soma and Batra, Amla "Ethno-medico-botany of household remedies of Phagi tehsil of Jaipur district

(Rajasthan)." *Ethnobotany,* Vol. 9, No. 1-2, 1997, pp. 122-128.

1598. Sen, Soma, Batra, Amla and Ali, Zulfikar Deewan "Some herbal home remedies from Jaipur district, Rajasthan". *Ethnobotany,* Vol. 14, No. 1-2, 2002, pp. 116-122.

1599. Sen, Sunil Kumar and Behera, Lalit Mohan "Ethnomedicinal plants used in touch therapy at Bargarh district of Orissa". *Ethnobotany,* Vol. 19, No. 1-2, 2007, pp. 100-104.

1600. Sen, Tulika "The health-status of the residual Andamanese". In Tribal Health edited by Buddhadeb Chaudhuri, New Delhi Inter India Publications, 1986.

1601. Sengupta, N. K. "Uncommon disease among adibasis (Ho) in Singhbhum district, Bihar". *Man in India,* Vol. 64, 1984, pp. 82-87.

1602. Sengupta, S. "Tree symbols worship in India" India Publishers, Calcutta, 1965.

1603. Senthilkumar, M., Gurumoorthi, P. and Janardhanan, K. "Some medicinal plants used by Irular, the tribal people of Marudhamalai hills, Coimbatore, Tamil Nadu". *Indian Journal of Natural Products and Resources,* Vol. 5, No. 5, 2006, pp. 382-388.

1604. Shah, A., Mukhopadhyay, S. B. and Gupta, D. Das "Inventory of indigenous healthcare practices of dairy animals". *Indian Journal of Traditional Knowledge,* Vol. 9, No. 2, 2009, pp. 326-332.

1605. Shah, G. L. and Gopal, G. V. "Folklore medicines of Vasavas, Gujarat, India". *Acta Botanica Indica,* Vol. 14, 1986, pp. 48-53.

1606. Shah, G.L., Menon, A.R. & Gopal, G.V. "An account of the ethnobotany of Saurashtra in Gujarat state". *Journal of Economic and Taxonomic Botany,* Vol. 2, 1981, pp. 173-182.

1607. Shah, G. L., Yadav, S. S. and Badri, N. "Medicinal plants from Dahanu forest division in Maharashtra state". *Journal of Economic and Taxonomic Botany,* Vol. 4, 1983, pp. 141-151.

1608. Shah, N. C. "Conservation of wild medicinal plants: need for a comprehensive strategy endangered species". *Kurukshetra*, Vol. 46, No. 3, 1997, pp. 15-17 and 33.

1609. Shah, N. C. "Endangered medicinal and aromatic taxa of U.P. Himalaya". In An Assessment of Threatened Plants of India, edited by S. K. Jain & R. R. Rao, 1983, pp. 40-49.

1610. Shah, N. C. "Ethnobotany and Indigenous Knowledge in Indian Context". *Ethnobotany,* Vol. 17, No. 1-2, 2005, pp. 64-70.

1611. Shah, N. C. "Ethnobotany in the Mountain Region of Kumaun Himalaya". Ph. D. Thesis (Unpublished). Kumaun University, Nainital, 1987.

1612. Shah, N. C. "Ethnobotany of some well known Himalayan Compositae". In Procedings of the International Compositae Conference, New Biology and Utilization, Royal Botanical Gardens, Kew. 1994, pp. 415-123.

1613. Shah, N. C. "Ethnographical and ethnomedicinal studies of Ladakh". *Ethnobotany,* Vol. 22, No. 1-2, 2010, pp. 73-81.

1614. Shah, N. C. "Herbal folk medicines in Northern India". *Journal of Ethnopharmacology*, Vol. 6, 1982, pp. 293-301.

1615. Shah, N.C. "Medicinal and aromatic plants in relation to the ecology of the mountainous region in the Kumaun Himalaya". In Science and Rural Development in Mountains edited by J. S. Singh et al., Gyanodhya Publication, Nainital. 1980, pp. 365-385.

1616. Shah, N.C. "Medico-botany of Dronagiri-The mythic hill in Kumaun (U.P.)". *Journal of Research in Indian Medicine*, Vol. 8, No. 1, 1971, pp. 47-59.

1617. Shah, N. C. "Need of systematic cultivation of medicinal herbs used in indigenous systems traditional medicine". *Indian drugs*, Vol. 18, No. 6, 1981, pp. 210-217.

1618. Shah, N. C. "Rauvolfia Serpentina: from folk-medicine to modern medicine-some unknown aspects". *Ethnobotany,* Vol. 7, No. 1-2, 1995, pp. 109-112.

1619. Shah, N. C. "The alpine medicinal herbs". *Indian Drugs*, Vol. 6, 1968, pp. 13-16.

1620. Shah, N. C. "The role of ethnobotany in relation to

medicinal plants in India". In Glimpses of Indian Ethnobotany edited by S. K. Jain, New Delhi, Oxford and IBH, 1981, pp. 69-80.

1621. Shah, N. C. and Gupta, L. K. "Useful medicinal plants of Ranikhet-I". *Indian Drugs*, Vol. 14, 1976, pp. 47-52.

1622. Shah, N. C. and Jain, S. K. "Ethnomedicobotany of Kumaun Himalaya, India". *Social Pharmacol*, Vol. 2, 1980, pp. 359-380.

1623. Shah, N. C. and Joshi, M. C. "An ethnobotanical study of Kumaun region of India". *Economic Botany*, Vol. 25, No. 4, 1971, pp. 414-422.

1624. Shah, N. C. and Kapoor, L. D. "Depletive medicinal plants of Kumaun Himalaya". *Journal of Research in Indian Medicine and Homoeopathy,* Vol. 13, pp. 38-43.

1625. Shah, Rohita, Pande, P. C. and Tiwari, Lalit "Traditional veterinary herbal medicines of western part of Almora district Uttarakhand Himalaya". *Indian Journal of Traditional Knowledge,* Vol. 7, No. 2, 2008, pp. 355-359.

1626. Shahu, Chaturbhuj "Indigenous knowledge of herbal treatment among the tribes of Hazaribagh district, Jharkhand". In Tribes and their indigenous knowledge: implications for development, edited by S. N. Chaudhary, IGRMS, Bhopal and Pratibha Prakashan, Delhi, 2008, pp. 138-146.

1627. Shalini, Kumari "Vedic leguminous plants: medicinal and microbiological study". New Delhi, Classical Publishing, 1997, p. 96.

1628. Shanavaskhan, A. E., Sivadasan, M. Alfarhan, Ahmad H. and Thomas, Jacob H. "Ethnomedicinal aspects of angiospermic epiphytes and parasites of Kerala, India". *Indian Journal of Traditional Knowledge,* Vol. 11, No. 2, 2012, pp. 250-258.

1629. Shankar, D. S. "Revitalizing local health traditions". In Food for thought: ancient visions and new experiments of rural people, edited by B. Haverkort and Wim Hiemstra, London, Zed Books, 1999, pp. 43-51.

1630. Shankar, Darshan "Cultural cross, current tribal medicine, ayurveda and modern medicine in the context of primary health care: A balanced view". *Ancient Science of Life,* Vol. 5, No. 2, 1985, pp.81-85.

1631. Shankar, Darshan "Indigenous Health Services-The State of the Art". In State of India's Health, edited by A. Mukhopadhyay, New Delhi, Voluntary Health Association of India, 1992, pp.129-162.

1632. Shankar, Darshan, Unnikrishnan, P. M. and Venkatasubramanian, Padma "Need to develop inter-cultural standards for quality, safety and efficacy of traditional Indian systems of medicine". *Current Science*, Vol. 92, No. 11, 2007, pp. 1499-1505.

1633. Shankar, Rama and Rawat, M.S. "Medicinal plants uses in traditional medicine in Lonit and Dibang valley district of Arunachal pradesh". *Indian Journal of Traditional Knowledge,* Vol. 7, No. 2, 2008, pp. 288-295.

1634. Shankara, M.R. "Folklores collected from traditional vaidyas". *Nagarjun*, Vol. 23, No.1, 1979, pp. 9-12.

1635. Shankara, M.R., Venkataram, B. S. and Leelavathy, S. "A 19th century manuscript on traditional medicine". *Bulletin of Indian Institute of History of Medicine*, Vol. 9, 1979, 33-37.

1636. Sharief, M.U. "Plants folk medicine of Negrito tribes of bay Islands". *Indian Journal of Traditional Knowledge,* Vol. 6, No. 3, 2007, pp. 468-476.

1637. Sharma, A.N. "An appraisal of folk medicines for the cure of diabetes among Bharias of Patalkot (M.P.) India". *Indian Journal of Physical Anthropology and Human Genetics,* Vol. 2, No. 2, 2004, pp. 247-251.

1638. Sharma, A. N. "Ethno-medicine used for the cure of drophobia among aboriginals of patalkot, Madhya Pradesh, India". *Madhya Bharati*, Vol. 43, No. 1, 1999, pp. 67-72.

1639. Sharma, Anima "Health and hygiene among the tribals: A case of Gonds". *The Anthropologist*, Vol. 3, No. 3, 2001, pp. 191-194.

1640. Sharma, Awadesh N. and Gautam, Rajesh K., Gharami, Ajay K. "Indigenous health care and ethno-medicine". New Delhi, Sarup & Sons, 2006, p. 295.

1641. Sharma, B.D. and Malhotra, S.K. "Contribution to the

ethnobotany of tribal area in Maharashtra". *Journal of Economic and Taxonomic Botany*, Vol. 5, 1984, pp. 533-537.

1642. Sharma, B. N. "Melghat kshetra ki Pramparagat Vanaushadhiyan: Melghat ke Korku aadivasiyo dwara prayukt aushadhi- Vidhiyan". *Vanyajati*, Vol. 43, No. 4, 1995, pp. 30-34. [Hindi]

1643. Sharma, Devinder "Digital library on Indian medicine systems: Another tool biopiracy". *Economic and Political Weekly,* Vol. 37, No. 25, 2002, 2416-2417.

1644. Sharma, Himanshu and Ashwani Kumar "Ethnobotanical studies on medicinal plants of Rajasthan (India): A review". *Journal of Medicinal Plants Research*, Vol. 5, No. 7, pp. 1107-1112.

1645. Sharma, K.N. "How the Uthlu-Birhor makes their living". *Vanyajati*, Vol. 6, 1958, pp. 173-176.

1646. Sharma, L. and Khandelwal, S. "Traditional uses of plants as cooling agents by the Tribal and Traditional communities of Dang region in Rajasthan, India". *Ethnobotanical Leaflets*, Vol. 14, 2010, pp. 218-224.

1647. Sharma, Laxmi Kant and Ashwini Kumar "Traditional medicinal practices of Rajasthan". *Indian Journal of Traditional Knowledge,* Vol. 6, No. 3, 2007, pp. 531-533.

1648. Sharma, Laxmi Kant, Dadhic, N. K. and Ashwani Kumar "Plant based veterinary medicine from traditional knowledge of India". *Bulletin of the Botanical Survey of India*, Vol. 47, 2005, pp. 1-4.

1649. Sharma, Laxmikant, Agarwal, Gaurav and Kumar, Ashwani "Medicinal plants for skin and hair care". *Indian Journal of Traditional Knowledge,* Vol. 2, No. 1, 2003, pp. 62-68.

1650. Sharma, Leena and Khandelwal, Sitaram "Weeds of Rajasthan and their ethno-botanical importance". *Studies on Ethno- medicine*, Vol. 4, No. 2, 2010, pp. 75-79.

1651. Sharma, N. K. "Ethnomedicine of Gadolia Lohars of Rajasthan". *Zoo's Print Journal*, Vol. 16, No. 9, 2001, pp. 593-594.

1652. Sharma, Neeta "Medicinal Use of Macro Fungi". *Ethnobotany,* Vol. 15, No. 1-2, 2003, pp. 97-99.

1653. Sharma, Neetu "Indigenous medication used by Himachali women to cure pregnancy discomforts". *Indian Journal of Traditional Knowledge,* Vol. 7, No. 4, 2008, pp. 638-641.

1654. Sharma, P. C. "Folk-lore antifertility plant drug of Bihar". *Bulletin of Medico-Ethno-Botanic Research*, Vol. 2, 1981, pp. 296-302.

1655. Sharma, P. C. and Sinha, G. N. "Folklore medicinal plants of Rachi (Bihar)". *Nagarjun*, Vol. 24, No. 1, 1980, pp. 1-6.

1656. Sharma, P.C., Murthy, K.S., Bhat, A.V., Narayanappa, D., Kishore, P. "Medicinal-lore of Orissa-1, Skin disease". *Bulletin of Medico-ethno-Botanical Research*, Vol. 6, 1985, pp. 93-101.

1657. Sharma, P. Dash and Sen, Pravir Kumar "Conservation of biodiversity in Mandar (Ranchi, Bihar): A Preliminary survey". *South Asian Anthropologist*, Vol. 16, No. 2, 1995, pp. 85-94.

1658. Sharma, P. P. and Mujumdar, A. M. "Traditional knowledge on plants from Toranmal plateau of Maharashtra". *Indian Journal of Traditional Knowledge,* Vol. 2, No. 3, 2003, pp. 292-296.

1659. Sharma, P.P. and Singh, N.P. "Ethnomedicinal Uses of some edible plants in Dadra, Nagar Haveli and Daman (U.T.)". *Ethnobotany*, Vol. 13, No. 1-2, 2001, pp. 121-125.

1660. Sharma, P. P. and Singh, N. P. "Less-known Ethnobotanical uses of Plants in Dadra & Nagar Haveli: (U.T): Part I (A-K)". *Ethnobotany*, Vol. 11, No. 1-2, 1999, pp. 109-114.

1661. Sharma, P. P. and Singh, N. P. "Less-known Ethnobotanical uses of Plants in Dadra and Nagar Haveli: (U.T.): part II (L-Z)". *Ethnobotany*, Vol. 12, No. 1-2, 2000, pp. 81-85.

1662. Sharma, P.V. "Indian medicine in the classical age". Varanasi, Chowkhamba Sanskrit Series Office, 1972, p. 265.

1663. Sharma, P.V, Murthy, K.S., Bhat, A.V., Narayanappa, D. and Kishore, P. "Medicinal folklore of Orissa-II. Gastrointestinal disorders". *Bulletin of Medico-ethno-botanical Research,* Vol. 7, 1986, pp. 26-40.

1664. Sharma, Parveen Kumar, Chauhan, N. S. and Lal, Brij

"Studies on plant assoiated indigenous knowledge among the Malanis of Kullu district, Himachal Pradesh". *Indian Journal of Traditional Knowledge,* Vol. 4, No. 4, 2005, pp. 403-408.

1665. Sharma, Parveen Kumar, Sethi, G.S. and Sharma, S.K. "Ethnomedicinal observations among the inhabitants of cold desert area of Himachal Pradesh". *Indian Journal of Traditional Knowledge,* Vol. 5, No. 3, 2006, pp. 358-361.

1666. Sharma, Poonam and Sharma, Jayashri Devi "Ethnomedicine in India and an approach towards medicinal ecology". *Bulletin of Medico-Ethno-Botanical Research,* Vol. 20, No. 1-4, 1999, pp. 1-19.

1667. Sharma, R.K., Dhyani, S.K. and Shankar, V. "Some useful and medicinal plants of the district Dehra Dun and Siwalik". *Journal of Science Research Plant Medicine,* Vol. 1, 1979, pp. 17-43.

1668. Sharma, R., Adhikari, D. and Majumder, M. "Traditional medicobotany of chakma community residing in the northwestern periphery of Namdapha national park in Arunachal pradesh". *Indian Journal of Traditional Knowledge,* Vol. 7, No. 4, 2008 pp. 587-593.

1669. Sharma, Ravindra "Medical Plants of India: An Encyclopaedia". Delhi, Daya Publishing House, 2003.

1670. Sharma, S. "The system of Ayurveda". Delhi, Neeraj Publishing House, 1923.

1671. Sharma, S.C. "Traditional herbal medicines from Shahjahanpur district, Uttar Pradesh - I". *Vegetos* Vol. 4, No. 1/2, 1991, pp. 76-80.

1672. Sharma, S.C. "Traditional herbal medicines from Shahjahanpur district, Uttar Pradesh — II". *Vegetos* Vol. 6, No. 1/2, 1993, pp. 9-14.

1673. Sharma, U.K., "Folk and herbal medicine among Nepalese of Assam". In Ethnobotany and medicinal plant of Indian subcontinent, edited by J.K. Maheshwari, Saujanya Books, Jodhpur, 2003, p. 672.

1674. Sharma, Ursula "Contextualizing alternative medicine". *Anthropology Today*, Vol. 9, No. 1-6, 1993, pp. 15-17.

1675. Sharma, Y.K. "Ayurveda in Rajtrangni-Kalahana's treatise of ancient Kashmir". *Indian Journal of Traditional Knowledge,* Vol. 6, No. 4, 2007, pp. 600-662.

1676. Sharpe, Elizabeth (ed.) "Eight-hundred year old book of Indian medicine and formulas". New Delhi, Asian Educational Services, 1979, p. 135.

1677. Shashikanth, J., Reddy, P. Ramachandra and Rao, P. Padma "Some indigenous folklore animal health care practices from Nalgonda district, Andhra Pradesh". *Ethnobotany,* Vol. 23, No. 1-2, 2011, pp. 78-81.

1678. Shawl, Humaira Yousuf, Tripathi, Laxmi and Bhattacharya, S. "Antidiabetic plants used by tribals in Madhya Pradesh". *Indian Journal of Natural Products and Resources,* Vol. 3, No. 6, 2004, pp. 75-82.

1679. Shekhawat, Dikha and Batra, Amla "Ethnobotany of some Household Remedies used against Animal and Insect Bite in Bundi district, Rajasthan". *Ethnobotany,* Vol. 18, No. 1-2, 2006, pp. 131-134.

1680. Sheldon, J.W., Balick, M.J. and Laird, S.A. "Medicinal plants: cn utilization and conservation coexist?". *Economic Botany*, Vol. 12, 2000, pp. 1-104.

1681. Shivanna, M.B. and Rajakumar, N. "Ethno- medico-botanical knowledge of rural folk in Bhadravathi taluk of Shimoga district, Karnataka". *Indian Journal of Traditional Knowledge,* Vol. 9, No. 1, 2010, pp. 158-162.

1682. Shivaprasad, B. and Chandrashekar, K.R. "Production of ayurvedic medicine in Dakshina Kannada district of coastal Karnataka". *Indian Journal of Traditional Knowledge,* Vol. 2, No. 3, 2003, pp. 272-283.

1683. Shome, Usha and Mehrotra, Shanta "Pharmacognostic Studies on 'Dronpushpi'". *Ethnoboatny*, Vol. 2, No. 1-2, 1990, pp. 105-115.

1684. Shosh, D.M. Anantharaman and Shetty, D.M.V. "Antifertility activity of an indigenous medicine 'Laksha'". *Bulletin of Medico-ethno-Botany Research*, Vol. 1, 1980, pp. 107-113.

1685. Shrivastava, A.K. "Technology road map for herbals as renewable bioresources and tribal health care". In Tribal health and medicines, edited by A. K. Kalla and P. C. Joshi, New Delhi, Concept Publishing Co., 2004, pp. 343-350.

1686. Shrivastava, J.L., Jain, Seema and Dubey, Abhilasha "Ethno-medicine for anti-fertility used by the tribals in Bastar district of Madhya Pradesh". In Ethnobotany and medicinal plant of Indian subcontinent, edited by J.K. Maheshwari, Saujanya Books, Jodhpur, 2003, p. 672.

1687. Shrivastava, Sushmita, Jain, Ashok Kumar and Mathur, R. "Documentation of herbal medicines used in treatment of disease of goats (cypris communis) in and arund Gwalior". *Indian Journal of Natural Products and Resources*, Vol. 3, No. 2, 2012, pp. 278-280.

1688. Shukla, Ajay Kumar and Bajpayee, Kaptain K. "Study of some uncommon folk medicial plants of Hardoi district (U.P.) India". *Vanyajati*, Vol. 58, no. 1, 2010, pp. 21-23.

1689. Shukla, B. R. K. "Drinks and drugs in a North India village-an anthropological study". Lucknow, Ethnographic Folk Culture Society, 1983.

1690. Shukla, Gyanesh and Verma, B. K. "Roots—a vital plant part to cure body ailments among tribal/rural folklore of Western Bihar". In Ethnobotany and medicinal plants of Indian sub-continent, edited by J. K. Maheshwari, Jodhpur, India Scientific Publishers, 2000.

1691. Shukla, K. P. "Traditional healers in community health". Gomati Krishna Publications, Varanasi, 1980.

1692. Shukla, P. R. "Moghiya Adivasi: deshi jadi bootiyo ke vishesagya (Adim chikitsa Vyavastha ka Samaj Sastriya Addhyan)". *Vanyajati*, Vol. 39, No. 2, 1991, pp. 13-24.

1693. Shukla, Rajesh and Chakravarty, Moyna "Study of traditional medicinal practices among the Raj-Gonds of Korba district of Chhattisgarh". *Studies on Ethno-medicine,* Vol. 4, No. 4, 2010, pp. 211-216.

1694. Shukla, Rajesh, Chakravarty, Moyna and Gautam, M.P. "Indigenous medicine used for treatment of gynaecological disorders by tribal of Chhattisgarh, India". *Journal of Medicinal Plants Research*, Vol. 2, No. 12, December, 2008, pp. 356-360.

1695. Shukla, S.P. "Indigenous drugs and their utilization by human beings". *Nagarjun*, Vol. 29, No. 5, 1986, pp. 10-11.

1696. Shukla, Shailesh and Gardner, James "Local knowledge

in community-based approaches to medicinal plant conservation: lessons from India". *Journal of Ethnobiology and Ethnomedicine*, Vol. 2, No. 20, 2006. (http://www.ethnobiomed.com/content/5/1/10)

1697. Shyamsunder and Parameshwarappa, P. S. "Non-wood forest products and tribal medicine". *My Forest*, Vol. 26, No. 4, 1990, pp. 387-395.

1698. Siddiqi, Muhammad Zubayr "Studies in Arabic and Persian Medical literature". Calcutta, Calcutta University, 1959, p. 173.

1699. Sidhu, Kiranjot and Pannu, Kunwarjeet "Indigenous use of medicinal plants for health care". *Studies on Ethnomedicine*, Vol. 4, No. 2, 2010, pp. 145-148.

1700. Sidu, Kiranjot, Kaur, Jasjeet and Kumar, Gurvinder "Prevention and cure of digestive disorders through the use of medicinal plants". *Journal of Human Ecology*, Vol. 21, No. 2, 2007, pp. 113-116.

1701. Sikarwar, R.L.S. "A brief account of Plants of Ramcharitmanas: a sacred book of Hindus". *Ethnobotany,* Vol. 5, No. 1-2, 1993, pp.155-159.

1702. Sikarwar, R.L.S. "Ethnomedicine of North Surguja forest division, Ambikapur, M.P.". *Aaryavaidyan*, Vol. 6, No. 2, 1992, pp. 97-100.

1703. Sikarwar, R.L.S., Pathak, Bharat and Jaiswal, Anil "Some unique Ethnomedicine perceptions of tribal communities of chitrakoot, Madhya pradesh". *Indian Journal of Traditional Knowledge,* Vol. 7, No. 4, 2008, pp. 613- 617.

1704. Sikdar, Mithun and Dutta, Uzzal "Traditional phytotherapy among the Nath people of Assam". *Studies on Ethnomedicine,* Vol. 2, No. 1, 2008, pp. 39-45.

1705. Sil, Arun K. "Total and integral medicine". Calcutta, Siva International Society for Creative Consciousness, 1994, p. 148.

1706. Silja, V.P. and Varma, K. Samitha "Ethnomedicinal plant knowledge of the Mullu Kuruma tribe of Wayanad district, Kerala". *Indian Journal of Traditional Knowledge,* Vol. 7, No. 4, 2008, pp. 604-612.

1707. Silkarwar, R.L.S. "Ethnogynaecological Uses of Plants new to India". *Ethnobotany,* Vol. 14, No. 1-2, 2002, pp. 112-115.

1708. Silori, Chandra Shekhar and Rana, Avnish R. "Indigenous knowledge on medicinal plants and their Narayan Sarovar Sanctuary, Kachchh". *Ethnobotany*, Vol. 12, No. 1-2, 2000, pp. 1-7.

1709. Singh, Giyan, Singh, H. B. and Mukherjee, T.K. (ed.) "Ethnomedicine of North-East India". New Delhi, NISCAIR, 2003.

1710. Singh, N., Swami, A., Gupta, B.K. and Grover, S.P. "Some noteworthy medicinal plants of commercial potential of Doon valley". *Indian Journal of Physical and Natural Sciences*, Vol. 9, April, 1993, pp. 24-33.

1711. Singh, P. Kumar and Singh, H.B. Kumar "Superstition in botanical folklore with reference to Meitei culture". In Ethnobotany and medicinal plants of Indian Sub-continent, edited by J.K. Maheshwari, Jodhpur, India Scientific Publishers, 2000.

1712. Singh, V. and Pandey, R.P. "Medicinal plant lore of the tribals of East Rajasthan". *Journal of Economic and Taxonomic Botany,* Vol. 1, 1980, pp. 137-147.

1713. Singh, A. K. "The myth of the healthy tribal report of ICMR task-force on Health Moderning Education Project (HMEP)" P.G. Department of Psychology, Ranchi University, Ranchi, 1987.

1714. Singh, A. K. "The Myth of the healthy tribal". *Social Change*, March, Vol. 17, No.1, 1987, pp. 3-23.

1715. Singh, A.P. "Healing practices among the tribes of Uttaranchal". In Tribal health and medicines, edited by A.K. Kalla and P.C. Joshi, New Delhi: Concept Publishing Co., 2004, pp. 242-246.

1716. Singh, A.P. "Concepts of disease and healing among the folk cultures of Uttaranchal Himalaya". *The Oriental Anthropologist*, Vol. 2, No., 2002, pp. 51-54.

1717. Singh, Ajay "Plants in Ancient Indian Civilizations". Delhi, Agam Kala Prakashan, 2008, p. 330.

1718. Singh, Ajit K. "Forest and tribal in India". New Delhi, Classical Publication Company, 1998, p. 176.

1719. Singh, Anamika, Singh, Ranjay K. and Sureja, Amish K. "Cultural significance and diversities of ethnic foods of

Northeast India". *Indian Journal of Traditional Knowledge,* Vol. 6, No. 1, 2007, pp. 79-94.

1720. Singh, Anand "Use of indigenous knolwedge and social networking in resource management: A case study in sustainable development from Kwazulu-natal". *Journal of Social Science*, Vol 4, No. 1, 2000.

1721. Singh, Brahma, O.P. Chaurasia and K.L. Jadhav "An ethnobotanical study of Indus Valley (Ladakh)". In Ethnobotany and medicinal plants of Indian Sub-continent, edited by J.K. Maheshwari, Jodhpur, India Scientific Publishers, 2000.

1722. Singh, G. and Kachroo, P. "Forest Flora of Srinagar". Bishan Singh Mahendra Pal Singh, Dehradun, 1976.

1723. Singh, Gajendra and Rawat, G.S. "Ethnomedicinal survey of Kedarnath Wildlife Sanctuary in Western Himalaya, India". *Indian Journal of Fundamental and Applied Life Sciences,* Vol. 1, No. 1, 2011, pp. 35-46.

1724. Singh, G.S., Saxena, K.G. and Rao, K.S. "Traditional knowledge and threat of its extinction in Chhakinal watershed in north western Himalaya". *Man in India,* Vol. 76, No. 1, 1996, pp. 1-17.

1725. Singh, Gopal S. "A Contribution to Ethnomedicine of Alwar district of Rajasthan". *Ethnoboatny*, Vol. 11, No. 1-2, 1999, pp. 97-99.

1726. Singh, Gopal S. "Functional attributes of tribal people of western Himalaya: Need for indigenous knowledge based sustainable planning". *Journal of Human Ecologist*, Vol. 17, No. 4, 2005, pp. 307-312.

1727. Singh, Gopal S. "Indigenous knowledge and conservation practices in tribal society of western Himalaya: A case study of Sangla Valley". *Studies of Tribes and Tribals,* Vol. 2, No. 1, 2004, pp. 29-35.

1728. Singh, H. "Ethnobiological treatment of piles by Bhoxas of Uttar Pradesh". *Ancient Science of Life*, Vol. 8, 1988, pp. 167-170.

1729. Singh, H. and Maheshwari, J. K. "Phytotherapy for Diphtheria by the Bhoxas of Nainital District, Uttar Pradesh, India". *Ethnobotany,* Vol. 5, 1993, pp. 63-65.

1730. Singh, H. and Maheshwari, J. K. "Traditional remedies for Snake-bite and scorpion sting among the Boxas of Nainital district, U.P.". *Aryavaidyan*, Vol. 6, No. 2, 1992, pp. 120-123.

1731. Singh, H. B. "Herbal Medicine of Manipur: A colour encyclopaedia". Delhi, Daya Publishing House, 2003, p. 77.

1732. Singh, H. B. "Plants used in medico-sexual purposes by the Meitei community in Manipur state, India". *Journal of Economic and Taxonomic Botany, Add. Series*. No. 12, 1996, pp. 364-366.

1733. Singh, H. B. "Studies on medico-botany of Meitei community in Manipur state, India III". *Advances in Plant Sciences,* Vol. 9, No. 2, 1997, pp. 27-30.

1734. Singh, H. B. "Studies on medico-botany of Meitei community in Manipur state, India II". *Advances in Plant Sciences*, Vol. 9, No. 2, 1997, pp. 13-18,

1735. Singh, H. B. and Singh, Brojendro "Plants used for making traditional rosaries in Manipur". *Indian Journal of Traditional Knowledge,* Vol. 4, No. 1, 2005, pp. 15-20.

1736. Singh, H.B. and Sundriyal, R.C. "Common spices and their use in traditional medicinal system of ethnic groups of Manipur state, North eastern India". *Indian Journal of Traditional Knowledge,* Vol. 2, No. 2, 2003, pp. 148-158.

1737. Singh, H.B. and Viswanathan, M.V. "Useful pteridophytes of India-a gift of nature to human beings". In Ethnobotany in South Asia edited by J.K. Maheshwari, New Delhi, Scientific Publishers, 1996,

1738. Singh, H.B., Hynniewta, T. M. and Bora, P. J. "An Ethnobotanical note on wild edible plants of Tripura, India". *Ethnoboatny*, Vol. 11, No. 1-2, 1999, pp. 26-28.

1739. Singh, H.B., Hynniewta, T. M. and Bora, P. J. "Ethno-Medico-Botanical Studies in Tripura, India". *Ethnoboatny*, Vol. 9, No. 1-2, 1997, pp. 56-58.

1740. Singh, H.B., Singh, P. K. and Jain, A. "Ethno-biological studies in Manipur". *Journal of Hill Research*, Vol. 10, No. 1 1997, pp. 36-38.

1741. Singh, H.H. Bhagat "History of Hindoo medical science". New Delhi, Logos Press, 1998, p. 280.

1742. Singh, H., Saklani, A. and Lal, B. "Ethnobotanical observations on some Gymnosperms of Garhwal Himalaya, Uttar Pradesh India". *Economic Botany*, Vol. 44, 1990, pp. 349-354.

1743. Singh, Harish "Herbal recipes for spermatorrhoea by Bhoxa tribe of Uttaranchal". *Ethnobotany,* Vol. 15, No. 1-2, 2003, pp. 115-117.

1744. Singh, Harish "Some medicinal plants in Joshimath Block, District Chamoli-Garhwal". Ph. D. Theses, Garhwal University, Uttaranchal, 1986.

1745. Singh, Harish and Bisht, G.S. "Depletion of ethnomedicinal plants in Alpine region of Chamoli Garhwal along with concept of their conservation and multiplication". *Journal of Science Research Plant Medicine*, Vol. 9, No. 1 and 2, 1988, pp. 20-23.

1746. Singh, Harish and Maheshwari, J.K. "Phytotherapy for Diphtheria by the Bhoxas of Nainital District, Uttar Pradesh, India". *Ethnobotany,* Vol. 5, 1993, pp. 63-65.

1747. Singh, I. J. "A study of morbidity pattern in a rural community". *Health and Population Perspectives and Issues,* Vol. 2, No. 3, 1979, pp. 193-206.

1748. Singh, J., Bhuyan, T. C. and Ahmed, A. "Ethnobotanical studies on the mishing tribes of Assam with special reference to food and medicinal plants-I". In Ethnobotany and Medicinal Plants of Indian Sub-continent, edited by J.K. Maheshwari, Jodhpur, India Scientific Publishers, 2000.

1749. Singh, K.K. "Ethnobotanical studies of the Tharus of Kumaun region, Uttar Pradesh". In Ethnobotany of Kumaun Himalaya, edited by P.C. Pande, D.S. Pokharia and J. C. Bhatt, Scientific Publishers, Jodhapur, 1999, pp. 1-13.

1750. Singh, K.K. "Plants used against wound: a survey of Santhal medicine". *Journal of Indian Bot. Sociology* (abs.), 1989, pp. 104-105.

1751. Singh, K.K. and Anand Prakash "Observations on ethnobotany of the Kol tribe of Varanasi district, Uttar Pradesh, India". In Ethnobotany and medicinal plants of Indian Sub-continent, edited by J.K. Maheshwari, Jodhpur, India Scientific Publishers, 2000.

1752. Singh, K.K. and Kumar, Kaushal "Observations on Ethnoveterinary Medicine among the Gaddi Tribe of Kangra Valley, Himachal Pradesh". *Ethnobotany,* Vol. 12, No. 1-2, 2000, pp. 42-44.

1753. Singh, K.K. and Maheshwari, J.K. "Traditional Herbal Remedies among the Tharus of Bahraich district, U.P., India". *Ethnobotany,* Vol. 1, No. 1-2, 1989, pp. 51-56.

1754. Singh, K.K. and Maheshwari, J.K. "Traditional phytotherapy of some medicinal plants used by the Tharus of the Nainital district, Uttar Pradesh". *Pharmaceutical Biology*, Vol. 32, No. 1, 1994, pp. 51-58.

1755. Singh, K.K. and Prakash, Anand "Indigenous Phytotherapy among the Gond Tribe of Uttar Pradesh, India". *Ethnobotany,* Vol. 6, No. 1-2, 1994, pp. 37-41.

1756. Singh, K.K. and Singh, S.C. "Some medicinal plants in the folklore of Varanasi district, U. P.". *Bulletin of Medico-ethno-Botanical Research,* Vol. 6, 1985, pp. 28-34.

1757. Singh, K.K., and Maheshwari, J.K. "Forest in the life and economy of the tribals of Varansi district, U.P." *Journal of Economic and Taxonomic Botany*, Vol. 6, 1985, pp. 109-116.

1758. Singh, K.K., Palvi, S.K. & Singh, H.B. "Survey of some medicinal plants of Dharchula block in Pithoragarh district of Uttar Pradesh". *Bulletin of Medico-ethno-botanical Research,* Vol. 1, 1980, pp. 1-7.

1759. Singh, K.K., Prakash, Anand and Palvi, S.K. "Observations on some energy plants among the tribals of Madhya Pradesh". In Ethnobotany and medicinal plant of Indian subcontinent, edited by J. K. Maheshwari, Saujanya Books, Jodhpur, 2003, p. 672.

1760. Singh, K.K., S. Saha & J.K. Maheswari "Observation on the ethnobotany of Boxa tribe of Bajpur block of Nainital district, Uttar Pradesh". *Himalayan Research and Development,* Vol. 6, No. 1-2, 1987, pp. 25-29.

1761. Singh, K.P. and Chaturvedi, G.N. "Some traditional antidiarrhoeal drugs". *Nagarjun*, Vol. 25, No. 6, 1982, pp. 130-135.

1762. Singh, L.B., Singh, R.H. & Singh, R.S. "Scope of Indian medicine in primary health care". *Nagarjun*, Vol. 23, No. 11, 1980, pp. 236-238.

1763. Singh, M. P. "Indigenous medicinal plants, social forestry and tribals". Delhi, Daya Publishing House, 2003, p. 505.

1764. Singh, Madhu B. and Ranjana "Camel milk consumption pattern and its association with diabetes among Raika community of Jodhpur district of Rajasthan". *Studies on ethno-medicine*, Vol. 2, No. 2, 2008, pp. 103-105.

1765. Singh, N. K. and others "Trace elements of some selected medicinal plants of Manipur". *Indian Journal of Natural Products and Resources*, Vol. 1, No. 2, 2010, pp. 22-231.

1766. Singh, Nagendra Kr. "Vedic mythology". New Delhi, A. P. H. Publishing, 1997, p. 301.

1767. Singh, Neeta and Chauhan, S. V. S. "Studies on some Leaves (Patra) used for Worship in Brij Mandal". *Ethnobotany,* Vol. 16, No. 1-2, 2004, pp. 69-71.

1768. Singh, O.K. "Floristic study of Tamenglong district, Manipur with Ethnobotanical notes". Unpublished Ph.D. Thesis, Manipur University, 1991.

1769. Singh, P.K. and Singh, K.I. "Traditional alcoholic beverage, Yu of Meitei communities of Manipur". *Indian Journal of Traditional Knowledge,* Vol. 5, No. 2, 2006, pp. 184-190.

1770. Singh, P. Kumar, Elangbam, Vinita Devi and Huidrom, B.K. Singh "Ethnomedicinal studies of some plants used to enhance vocalism by the traditional meitei singers of Manipur". In Ethnobotany and medicinal plant of Indian subcontinent, edited by J.K. Maheshwari, Saujanya Books, Jodhpur, 2003, p. 672.

1771. Singh, Prabhat K. "Ethno - peasantry system: A case of the Kurmis". *Man in India,* Vol. 74, No. 2, 1994, pp. 169-179.

1772. Singh, R.S. and Singh, A.N. "On the identity and economic-medicinal use of Hasti Karnapalasa (Leea macrophylla Roxb, Fam. Ampelidaceae) as evinced in the ancient (Sanskrit) text and traditions". Indian *Journal of History of Science*, Vol. 16, 1981, pp. 219-222.

1773. Singh, Ram and Misri, Bimal "Traditional goat health management preactices in Chamba district of Himachal

Pradesh". *Indian Journal of Traditional Knowledge,* Vol. 5, No. 3, 2006, pp. 373-375.

1774. Singh, Ranjay K. "Learning the indigenous knowledge and biodiversity through contest: A participatory methodological tool of eco literacy". *Indian Journal of Traditional Knowledge,* Vol. 9, No. 2, 2010, pp. 355-360.

1775. Singh, Ranjay K. and Dwivedi, B. S. "An investigation into the indigenous knowledge for rainfall prediction". *Indian Journal of Traditional Knowledge,* Vol. 2, No. 2, 2003, pp. 181-188.

1776. Singh, Ranjay K. and Singh, Anamika "Women's wisdom and indigenous human healthcare practices". *Indian Journal of Traditional Knowledge,* Vol. 8, No. 2, 2009, pp. 262-269.

1777. Singh, Ranjay K. and Sureja, Amish K. "Centurion women and diverse knowledge systems". *Indian Journal of Traditional Knowledge,* Vol. 5, No. 3, 2006, pp. 413-419.

1778. Singh, Ranjit and Padmalatha, C. "Ethno-entomological practices in Tirunelveli district, Tamil Nadu". *Indian Journal of Traditional Knowledge,* Vol. 3, No. 4, 2004, pp. 442-446.

1779. Singh, S.K. and Rawat, G.S. "Traditional versus commercial use of wild medicinal plants of great Himalayan National Park". *Proceeding Mountain Meet,* No. 98, 1997.

1780. Singh, S.P. and Singh, V.L. "Folklore claims by tribals and experimental evaluation of some medicinal plants with special reference to contraception". In Tribal health: Socio-Cultural dimentions, edited by Buddhadeb Chaudhuri, New Delhi, Inter India, 1986, pp. 339-346.

1781. Singh, S.S. "Folk medicine of Manipur - The old traditional means of curing diseases". *Folklore,* Vol. 31, No. 1, 1990, pp. 7-13.

1782. Singh, Shweta, Dixit, R.D. and Sahu, T.R. "Ethnomedicinal uses of pteridophytes of Amarkantak, Madhya Pradesh". *Indian Journal of Traditional Knowledge,* Vol. 4, No. 4, 2008, pp. 392-395.

1783. Singh, Sumita "Kainsar nirodhak ausadhiya". *Yojana,* Vol. 35, No. 4, 1991, pp. 7-8.

1784. Singh, Sunil Kumar, Chaudhary, Anand and Rai, D.K. "Preparation and characterization of a mercury based Indian traditional drug-Ras-sindoor". *Indian Journal of Traditional Knowledge,* Vol. 8, No. 3, 2009, pp. 346-351.

1785. Singh, V. and Pandey, R.P. "Ethno-medicinal plants used for venereal and gynaecological diseases in Rajasthan (India)". In Ethnobotany and medicinal plants of Indian Sub-continent, edited by J.K. Maheshwari, Jodhpur, India Scientific Publishers, 2000.

1786. Singh, V.K. "Exploitation and threat to some medicinal plants and folk drugs of Garhwal and Kumaun regions of Uttar Pradesh, India". In Himalayan Biodiversity: Conservation Strategies edited by U. Dhar, Gyanodaya Prakashan, Nainital. 1992, pp. 107-412.

1787. Singh, V.K. "Some folklore medicines from district Subansiri of Arunachal Pradesh". *Bulletin of the Medico-ethno-Botanic Research,* Vol. 4, 1983 pp. 95-101.

1788. Singh, V.K., Ali, Z.A. and Siddiqui, M.K. "Ethnomedicine in the Bahraich district of Uttar Pradesh, India". *Fitoterapia* Vol. 67, No. 1, 1996, pp. 65-76

1789. Singh, V. K., Anis, M. & Khan, A. M. "Endangered medicinal plants of Chakrata forests, Uttar Pradesh, India". *Journal of Plants and Nature*, Vol. 1, 1984, pp. 36-40.

1790. Singh, V.P., Sharma, S.K. & Khare, V. S. "Medicinal Plants from Ujjain district Madhya Pradesh, Part II". *Indian Drugs pharm, Ind.* Vol. 15, No. 5, 1980, pp. 7-12.

1791. Singh, Vijay Pratap "Digital library to save tribal medicine from fake patents". (http://www.expressindia.com/latest-news/digital-library-to-save-tribal-medicine-from-fake-patents/317944/)

1792. Singh, Virendra and Chauhan, N.S. "Traditional practices of herbal medicines in the Lahaul valleys, Himachal Himalayas". *Indian Journal of Traditional Knowledge,* Vol. 4, No. 2, 2005, pp. 208-220.

1793. Singh, Yash K. "Folk medicines of the Mishings of Assam". *Vanyajati*, Vol. 49, No. 2, 2001, pp. 10-14.

1794. Singh, Udai Pratap "Tribal health in North East India: A study of socio-cultural dimensions of health care practices". New Delhi, Serials Publications, 2008, p. 182.

1795. Sinha, B.K. and Dixit, R.D. "Ethnobotanical Studies on Sarcostemma Acidum (Asclepiadaceae) from Khargaon district, Madhya Pradesh". *Ethnobotany,* Vol. 13, No. 1-2, 2001, pp. 116-117.

1796. Sinha, B.K. and Dixit, R.D. "Ethnomedicinal Plants sold in Omkareshwar, Madhya Pradesh". *Ethnobotany,* Vol. 15, No. 1-2, 2003, pp. 127-128.

1797. Sinha, B.K., Vinod Maina and P.M. Padhye "Ethnomedicinal plants of Bay Islands for skin care". In Ethnobotany and medicinal plants of Indian Sub-continent, edited by J.K. Maheshwari, Jodhpur, India Scientific Publishers, 2000.

1798. Sinha, Nirmal Kumar "Ayurveda: The traditional medicinal system of India with reference to medicine system of Birhors". *Vanyajati,* Vol. 57, No. 4, 2009, pp. 8-11.

1799. Sinha, R. and Sinha, Swetha "Renaissance of Traditional Herbal Medicine in India Fulfilling the Promise to Health for All in the 21 Century". *Curare,* Vol. 21, 1998, pp. 175-186.

1800. Sinha, R.K. "Anti-tumour activities of some traditional plants used by the mobile tribal medicine men (The street herbal vendors) in India". *Journal of Scientific Research in Plant Medicine,* Vol. 12, No. 3-4, 1991, pp. 40-42.

1801. Sinha, R.K. "Contribution of Indian Tribals to Modern Civilization". In Tribals in India: Development, Deprivation and Discontent edited by A.K. Kalla and P.C. Joshi, New Delhi: Har-Anand Publications, 1995, pp. 80-93.

1802. Sinha, R.L. "Protection and planned exploitation of Indian medicinal plants in the hills of Uttar Praedsh". In Proceeding of Natural Symposium on Recent Advance in the Dev. Prod. and Utilization of medicinal and aromatic plants, CIMAP, Lucknow. 24-26, Feb., 1975.

1803. Sinha, Rajiv K. "Anti tumour activities of some traditional plants used by the mobile tribal medicinemen (The street herbal vendors) in India". *Journal of Scientific Research in Plants and medicines,* Vol. 12, No. 3-4, 1991, pp. 40-42.

1804. Sinha, Rajiv K. "Ethnobiology: role of Indigenous and ethnic societies in biodiversity conservation, human health protection and sustainable development". Jaipur, Surabhi, 2001, p. 335.

1805. Sinha, Rajiv K. "Ethnobotany: the renaissance of traditional herbal medicine". Jaipur, INA Shree, 1996, p. 242.

1806. Sinha, Rajiv K. "Herbal remedies prescribed by the street herbal vendors (mobile tribal medicinemen) in the treatment of some common human ailments in India (Arthritis)". *Journal of Scientific Research in Plants and Medicine*, Vol. 11, No.1-4, 1989, pp. 36-42.

1807. Sinha, Rajiv K. "Herbal Remedies prescribed by the Street Herbal vendors (Tribal medicinemen) in the Treatment of some common human ecological disorders (Gynaecological disorders) in Women". *Ancient Science of Life*, Vol. 10, No. 3, 1991, pp. 207-210.

1808. Sinha, Rajiv K. "Legacy and ecology of the tribals: A gift to the modern civlization". In Indian Tribals, edited by R.C. Swarankar, Printwell Publishers, Jaipur, 1995.

1809. Sinha, Rajiv K. "Sustainable utilization and conservation of biodiversity by the tribal societies of India: A Lesson for modern man". *International Journal of Environmental Education and Information*, Vol. 14, No. 2, 1995.

1810. Sinha, Rajiv K. "Tribal Heritage: Their economic and ecological significance". In Studies in Tribal Development edited by G.P. Gupta, Vol. 1, 1991, Arihant Publisher., Jaipur. pp. 361-373.

1811. Sinha, Rajiv, K. "Conservation of cultural (ethnic) diversity of the indigenous people essential for protection of biological diversity". Proceedings of the 4th International Congress on Ethnobiology, Lucknow, Jaipur, 1994.

1812. Sinha, S.C. "Edible wild plants of Manipur". Report of workshop, Educational camp on environmental awareness, Manipur Peace Centre, 1986.

1813. Sinha, S.C. "Ethnomedicinal plants of Manipur and their conservation". Regional Seminar on medicinal plants, Ministry of Halth and Family Welfare, Govt. of India, 1986.

1814. Sinha, S.C. "Medicinal plants of Manipur". Imphal, Mass and Sinha, 1996, p. 238.

1815. Sinha, Surajit "Training of a Bhumij medicine-man". *Man in India,* Vol. 38, No. 2, 1958, pp. 111-128.

1816. Sinha, U.P. "Study of fertility of the Santals and the

Paharias of Santal Paraganas". *Bulletin of the Bihar Tribal Research Institute,* Vol. 5, No. 1, 1963, pp. 82-124.

1817. Sinha, U.P. "Traditional tribal medicine and modern health care system". In Tribal health in India, edited by Salil Basu, Delhi, Manak Publications, 1994, pp. 151-163.

1818. Siromoney, G.L., Giles, D. and Livingstone, C. "Herbal medicine of the Narikoravas". *Folklore*, Vol, 14, No. 10, 1973, pp. 363-366.

1819. Sivarajan, V.V. "Ayurvedic drugs and their plant sources". New Delhi, Oxford and IBH, 1994. p. 570.

1820. Sivaramakrishnan, Kavíta "Old potions, new bottles-Recasting indigenous medicine in colonial Punjab, 1850-1945". Orient Longman, New Delhi, 2006, p. 280.

1821. Solavan, A., Paulmurugan, R. and Wilsanand, V. "Antibacterial activity of subterranean termites used in South Indian folk medicine". *Indian Journal of Traditional Knowledge,* Vol. 6, No. 4, 2007, pp. 559-562.

1822. Solavan, A., Paulmurugan, R. and Wilsanand, V. "Effect of the subterranean termite used in the south Indian folk medicine". *Indian Journal of Traditional Knowledge,* Vol. 5, No. 3, 2006, pp. 376-379.

1823. Sonowal, Ripunjoy and Barua, Indira "Ethnomedical practices among the Tai-Khamyangs of Assam, India". *Studies on Ethno-medicine*, Vol. 5, No. 1, 2011, pp. 41-50.

1824. Sood, Shipra and Sharma, Avinash "Knowledge and urban homemakers in indigenous resource management practices". *Human Ecology*, Vol. 26, No. 2, 2009, pp. 85-87.

1825. Soumyanath, Amala (ed.) "Traditional medicines for modern times: antidiabetic plants". Taylor and Francis, 2005, p. 314.

1826. Sreenathan, M. "Language diversity, indigenous knowledge and biodiversity conservation: The symbiosis". *Journal of Social Anthropology*, Vol. 6, No. 1-2, 2009, pp. 1-10.

1827. Sri, B. Sandhya, and Reddi, T. V. V. Seetharami "Native herbal galactagogues used by women of Bagata tribe of Visakhapatnam district, Andhra Pradesh". *Ethnobotany,* Vol. 23, No. 1 and 2, 2011, pp. 125-128.

1828. Sri, B. Sandhya, Rao, J. Koteshwara and Reddi, T. V. V.

Seetharami "Plants used in magico-religious beliefs by the tribals of Visakhapatnam distrct, Andhra Pradesh". *Ethnobotany,* Vol. 23, No. 1-2, 2011, pp. 100-105.

1829. Sridevi, C. "Modern women, tribal medicine and social change". *Man and Life,* Vol. 15, No. 3-4, 1989, pp. 123-132.

1830. Srinivasa, B. M. "Ethno medical practices among the Jenu Kuruba of Karnataka". *Man and Life,* Vol. 36, No. 3-4, 2010, pp. 107-112.

1831. Srinivasan, Aruna "Alternative therapy". *Discover India,* Vol. 12, No. 4, 1999, pp. 32-34.

1832. Srinivasan, Padma "National health policy for traditional medicine in India". *World Health Forum,* Vol. 16, 1995, pp. 190-193.

1833. Srivasatava, R.C. and Nyishi Community "Traditional knowledge of Nishi (Dafla) tribe of Arunachal Pradesh". *Indian Journal of Traditional Knowledge,* Vol. 9, No. 1, 2010, pp. 26-27.

1834. Srivastava, Priya and Sahay, Vijoy S. "Traditional ecological knowledge vis-a-vis sustainable development in Sundarbans". *The Oriental Anthropologist,* Vol. 6, No. 1, 2006, pp. 192-199.

1835. Srivastava, R.C. and Adi Community "Traditional knowledge of Adi tribe of Arunachal Pradesh on plants". *Indian Journal of Traditional Knowledge,* Vol. 8, No. 2, 2009, pp. 146-153.

1836. Srivastava, R.C., Singh, Ranjay K. and Apatani Community "Indigenous biodiversity of Apatani plateau: Learning on bio-cultural knowledge of Apatani tribe of Arunachal Pradesh for sustainable livelihoods". *Indian Journal of Traditional Knowledge,* Vol. 9, No. 3, 2009, pp. 432-442.

1837. Srivastava, S.K. and Sekar, K. Chandra "Ethnomedicine of the Pin Valley National Park, Himachal Pradesh: Plants used in treating dysentery". *Ethnobotany,* Vol. 16, No. 1-2, 2004, pp. 62-63.

1838. Srivastava, T. N., Badola, D. P. & Gupta, O. P. "Medicinal herbs used by Amchies of Ladakh". *Bulletin of Medico-Ethno-Botanical Research,* Vol. 2, 1981, pp. 193-202.

1839. Srivastva, R. C. "Plant identity crisis in Indian systems of medicine". *Current Science,* Vol. 91, No. 9, 2006, p. 1125.

1840. Steiner, Richard P. "Folk medicine: The art and the science". American Chemical Society, 1986, p. 223.

1841. Stenson, Anthony J. and Gray, Tim S. "An autonomy-based justification for Intellectual Property Rights of indigenous communities". *Environmental Ethics*, Vol. 21, No. 2, 1999, pp. 177-190.

1842. Subba Rao, T.V. "Bamboo and its utilization". Indian Forest, Vol. 92, 1966, pp. 186-190.

1843. Subba Reddy, D.V. "The origin and growth of indigenous Unani medical literature in medieval India". *Indian Journal of History of Medicine*, Vol. 16, No. 1, 1969, p. 20.

1844. Subba, J.R. "Indigenous knowledge on bio- resources management for livelihood of the people of Sikkim". *Indian Journal of Traditional Knowledge,* Vol. 8., No. 1, 2009, pp. 56-64.

1845. Subbarayappa, B.V. (ed.) "Medicine and life sciences in India". New Delhi, Centre for Studies in Civilization/ Project of History of Indian Science, Philosophy and Culture 2001, p. 786.

1846. Subramanyam, Ragupathy, Newmaster, Steven G. and Paliyath, Gopinadhan "Exploring ethnobiological classifications for novel alternative medicine: A case of Cardiospermum halicacabum L. ('Modakathon', balloon vine) as a traditional herb for treating rheumatoid arthritis". *Ethnobotany*, Vol. 19, No. 1-2, 2007, pp. 1-16.

1847. Subramanyam, V. and Rao, P. Durga "Effect of deforestation in medicinal plants by the tribes of Visakha agency area, Andhra Pradesh". *South Asian Anthropologist*, Vol. 7, No. 2, 2007, pp. 167-171.

1848. Sud, Romesh Kumar "Herbs: Culinary, Medicinal, Aromatic (Secrets and Human happiness)". Jodhpur, Scientific Publishers, 2004, p. 273.

1849. Sudhakar, A., and Vedavathy, S. "Wild edible plants used by the tribals of Chittor district (Andhra Pradesh), India". In Ethnobotany and medicinal plant of Indian subcontinent, edited by J.K. Maheshwari, Saujanya Books, Jodhpur, 2003, p. 672.

1850. Sudhakar, S. and Rolla, R.S. "Medicinal plants of Upper

East Godavari district (Andhra Pradesh) and need for establishment of medicianl farm". *Journal of Economic and Taxonomic Botany,* Vol. 7, 1985, pp. 399-406.

1851. Sukumaran, S. and Raj, A. D. "Medicinal plants of sacred groves in Kanyakumari district Southern Western Ghats". *Indian Journal of Traditional Knowledge,* Vol. 9, No. 2, 2010, pp. 294-299.

1852. Sumitra, S. and Jamir, N.S. "Traditionally uses of medicinal plants used by Tangkhul- Naga Tribe in Manipur, India". *Pleione*, Vol. 3, No. 2, 2009, pp. 157-162.

1853. Sunanda, Mondal and Ranjan, Paul "Medicinal plants grown in and around Guskara used by local poor people for treating some common ailments". *Journal of Medicinal Plants Research,* Vol. 5, No. 19, 2011, pp. 4798-4803.

1854. Sundriyal, R.C., Negi, S.C., Joshi, A.P. and Dhasmana, R. "Some important medicinal trees of Kotdwara, lansdowne and vicinity". *Himalayan Chemistry Pharm. Bull.*, Vol. 2, 1985, pp. 45-48.

1855. Sur, P.R., Sen, R. Halder, A.C. and Bandyopadhyay, S. "Ethnomedicine in the Ayodhya hills region of the Purulia district, West Bengal, India". *Journal of Economic and Taxonomic Botany, Additional Series* 10, 1992, pp. 333-337.

1856. Suresh, K.P. "Indigenous agricultural practices among Mavilan tribe in North Kerala". *Studies of Tribes and Tribals,* Vol.8, No. 2, 2010, pp. 103-106.

1857. Suresh, Kuru, Senthilmurugan, G. Viji, Pandiselvam, P. Karuppuraja, S. "Ethnomedicinal plants used by the Rural people in Thiruppachethi village of Sivagangai District, Tamil Nadu, India". *Journal of Bioscience Research*, Vol. 3, No. 1, pp. 47-51.

1858. Susuman, A. Sathiya "Correlates Antenatal and postnatal care among tribal women in India". *Studies on Ethno-medicine*, Vol. 6, No. 1, 2012, pp. 55-62.

1859. Sutha, S., Mohan, V.R. and Kumaresan, S. "Ethnomedicinal plants used by the tribals of Kalakad-Mundanthurai tiger reserve (KMTR), Western Ghats, Tamil Nadu for the treatment of rheumatism". *Indian Journal of Traditional Knowledge,* Vol. 9, No. 3, 2010, pp. 502-509.

1860. Suthar, A. C., Banavalikar, M. M. and Biyani, M. K. "A review on ginger (Zingiber officinale): Pre-clinical and clinical tribals". *Indian Journal of Traditional Knowledge,* Vol.2, No. 1, 2003, pp. 51-61.

1861. Svoboda, Robert E. "Prakruti: your ayurvedic constitution". Delhi, Motilal Banarsidass, 1993. p. 206.

1862. Swamy, N. Satyanarayana and Reddi, T. V. V. Seetharami "Ethnomedicine for leucorrhoea from Adilabad district of Andhra Pradesh, India". *Ethnobotany,* Vol. 23, No. 1 and 2, 2011, pp. 147-149.

1863. Swanson, Timothy (ed.) "Intellectual property rights and biodiversity conservation: an interdisciplinary analysis of the values of medicinal plants". Cambridge, Cambridge University Press, 1995, p. 271.

1864. Syed, K.M.H. "Medicines among Gonds, Kolams and Chenchus". *Man in India,* Vol. 30, 1950, pp. 23-31.

1865. Tag, Hui and Das, A. K. "Ethnobotanical notes on the Hill Miri tribe of Arunachal Pradesh". *Indian Journal of Traditional Knowledge,* Vol. 3, No. 1, 2004.

1866. Tag, Hui, Das, A.K. and Kalita, Pallabi "Plants used by the hill miri tribe of Arunachal Pradesh in ethnofisheries". *Indian Journal of Traditional Knowledge,* Vol. 4, No. 1, 2005, pp. 57-64.

1867. Takhar, H.K. "Folk herbal veterinary medicines of southern Rajasthan". *Indian Journal of Traditional Knowledge,* Vol. 3, No. 4, 2004, pp. 407-418.

1868. Talukdar, Moromi "Beliefs and practices regarding disease and treatment among the Karbis of Assam". *The Oriental Anthropologist,* Vol. 2, No. 2, 2002, pp. 143-147.

1869. Tamsang K.P. "Glossary of Lepcha medicinal plants". Mani Printing Press, Kalimpong (West Bengal), India; 2004.

1870. Tamsang K.P. "The Unknown and Untold Reality about the Lepchas". Luen Sun Offset Printing Co. Hongkong, 1983.

1871. Tamuli, P. and Saikia, R. "Ethno-medico-botany of the zeme tribe of North Cachar hills district of Assam". *Indian*

Journal of Traditional Knowledge, Vol. 3, No. 4, 2004, pp. 430-436.

1872. Tamuli, P. and Sharma, P. "Ethno-medico-botany of the Dimasa Kachari of North Cachar Hills district of Assam". *Indian Journal of Traditional Knowledge*, Vol. 9, No. 4, 2010, pp. 718-770.

1873. Tanti, Bhaben and others "Assessment of antimicrobial and antioxidant activities of Dendrocnide sinuata (blume) chew leaves- A medicinal plants used by ethnic communities of Nort East India". *Indian Journal of Natural Products and Resources*, Vol. 1, No. 1, 2010, pp. 17-21.

1874. Tanti, Bhaben, Gurung, Lisha and Sarma, Hridip K. "Ethnobotany of starter cultures used in alcohol fermentation by a few ethnic tribes of Northeast India". *Indian Journal of Traditional Knowledge,* Vol. 9, No. 3, 2010, pp. 463-466.

1875. Tantray, Mudasir Ahmad and others "Ethnomedicinal survey of shopian, Kashmir (J&K), India". *Asian Journal of Traditional Medicines*, Vol. 4, No. 1, 2009.

1876. Tarafder, C.R. "Ethnobotany on Chhotonagpur: less known and unknown 38 medicinal plants used by the tribal". *Folklore*, Vol. 27, No. 6, 1986, pp. 119-125.

1877. Tarafder, C.R. "Less known nine medicinal plants used by the tribals for curing gonorrhoea in Ranchi and Hazaribagh districts, Bihar". *Folklore*, Vol. 25, 1984, pp. 47-49.

1878. Tarafder, C.R. "Less known twenty three medicinal plants used by the tribals for curing boils in Ranchi and Hazaribagh district, Bihar". *Vanyajati*, Vol. 32, 1984, pp. 14-19.

1879. Tarafder, C.R. "Some traditional knowledge about tribal health: plants used by the tribals of Haziribagh and Ranchi district". *Folklore*, Vol. 28, No. 2, 1987, pp. 37-42.

1880. Tarafder, C.R. "Traditional medicinal plants used by the tribals of Ranchi and Hazaribagh districts Bihar- Plants used in stomach trouble". *Journal of Economic and Taxonomic Botany*, Vol. 4, 1983, pp. 891-896.

1881. Tarafder, C.R. and Choudhury, H.N. Rai "Less known medicinal uses of plants among the tribals of Hazaribagh District, Bihar". In Glimpses of Indian Ethnobotany edited by S.K. Jain, New Delhi, Oxford and IBH, 1981, pp. 208-217.

1882. Tayung, Kumananda and Saikia, Nabin "Crytolepis buchanani- a less-known medicinal plant used in bone fracture". *Indian Journal of Traditional Knowledge,* Vol. 2, No. 4, 2003, pp. 371-374.

1883. Tewari, K.C. and others "Adulteration of Saffron (Crocus sativus Linn.) and its detection". Sachitra Ayurved, December 1995, pp. 635-637.

1884. Tewari, K.C., Joshi, G.C. and Uniyal, M.R. "Verbascum Thapsus Linn: highly bactericidal herb scabies from Kumoun Himalaya". *Sachitra Ayurved*, December 1989, pp. 400-410.

1885. Tewari, K.C., Joshi, G.C., Tewari, R.N. and Pandey, N.K. "Lobellia pyamidalis Wall: A drug for asthma from Himalayan folklore". *Sachitra Ayurved*, December, 1989, pp. 198-400.

1886. Tewari, K.C., Pandey, G.C., Pandey, N.K. and Tewar, K.C. "Some rare folk tribal medicines from Garo Hills in North Eastern India". *Journal of Economic and Taxonomic Botany*, Vol. 10, 1994, pp. 319-322.

1887. Tewari, K.C., Tewari, R.N. and Joshi, G.C. "Ayurvedic ausadhi virkasyan dwera vani karan (in Hindi)". *Sachitra Ayurved*, January 1990, pp. 399-405.

1888. Tewari, K.C., Tewari, R.N., Joshi, G.C. and Pandey, G. "Saving endangered medicinal plant resources of hills, Uttarakhand". Uttarakhand Sodha Sansthan, Pantnagar, 1992, pp. 84-90.

1889. Tewari, K.C., Tewari, R.N., Pant, S.C. and Joshi, G.C. "On the introduction of valuable medicinal plant from North Eastern to Western Himalayan region of India". *Bulletin of Medico-Ethno Botanical Research,* Vol. 14, No. 3-4, 1993, pp. 525-526.

1890. Tewari, L.C. and others "Some traditional folk medicines from the Himalayas (U.P. region)". *Aaryavaidyan*, Vol. 4, No. 1, 1990, pp. 49-57.

1891. Tewari, L.C., Sanwal, P., Singh, J., and Joshi, P. "Preliminary phytochemical screening of medicinal plants of hilly districts (Kumaun and Garhwal divisions) of U.P.". *Bulletin of Medico-Ethno Botanical Research,* Vol. 5, 1984, pp. 71-81.

1892. Tewari, V.P. and Joshi, P. "Tau-Dam practices of hill area of Uttar Pradesh". *CCRAS News letter*, Vol. 7, No. 6, 1983.

1893. Tewari, V.P., Tewari, K.C. amd Yadav, B.B. L. "Valeanana in India medicine vis-a-vis modern medicine". *Journal of Research in Indian Medicine,* Vol. 9, No. 4, 1974.

1894. Tewari, V.P., Tewari, K.C. Pandey, N.K. and Joshi, G. C. "Ausadh durpyog (Drug abuse) ke karan evem nira karan". *Sachitra Ayurved,* August, 1995, pp. 301-303.[Hindi]

1895. Thakur, G. C. S. "Ethno Medicine and Tribal Health". *Bulletin of the Department of Anthropology, Dibrugarh University,* Vol. 25, 2002, pp. 65-72.

1896. Thakur, Neeraj Kumar "The Saperas (snake charmers) of Shankargarh: A study in continuity and change of traditional knowledge and wisdom". In Traditional Knowledge in Contemporary Societies: Challenges and Apportunities, edited by Kamal K. Misra and K.K. Basa, IGRMS, Bhopal & Pratibha Prakashan, Delhi, 2007.

1897. Thakur, R.S., Puri, H.S. and Husain, A. "Major medicinal Plants of India". CIMAP, Lucknow, 1989.

1898. Thirumulpadu, Vaidyabhooshanam K. Raghavan "Ayurvedadarsanam (Malayalam)". Thiruvananthapuram, State Institute of Languages, 1997, p. 157.

1899. Thomas, Jery and Britto, A. John De "Weeds of medicinal importance in Tirunelveli district in Tamil Nadu". In Ethnobotany and medicinal plant of Indian subcontinent, edited by J. K. Maheshwari, Saujanya Books, Jodhpur, 2003, p. 672.

1900. Thothathri, K. "Interesting and useful plants of the Andaman and Nicobar Islands". *Indian Museum Bulletin,* Vol. 9, No. 2, 1974, pp. 26-28.

1901. Thothathri, K. "Plant resources and their utilization in the Andaman and Nicobar Islands". *Journal of Economic and Taxonomic Botany,* Vol. 1, 1980, pp. 111-114.

1902. Thottam, Paul Joseph "Siddha medicine: A handbook of traditional remedies". In Lives and deeds of the Siddhars (Penguin Books India, New Delhi), 2000, pp. 6-17.

1903. Tirkey, Amia "Some ethnomedicinal plants of family-Fabaceae of Chhattisgarh state". *Indian Journal of*

Traditional Knowledge, Vol. 5, No. 4, 2006, pp. 551-553.

1904. Tiwari, Ashok K. "Karela: A promising antidiabetic vegetable therapy". *Current Science*, Vol. 91, No. 9, 2006, pp. 1697-1701.

1905. Tiwari, Bal Govind and Upadhyay, B. N. "Concept of aging in ayurveda". *Indian Journal of Traditional Knowledge,* Vol. 8, No. 3, 2009, pp. 396-399.

1906. Tiwari, K.C. "Plants used in tribal medicine of Garo hills (Meghalaya)". *Sachitra Ayurved*, Vol. 48, No. 3, 1995, pp. 387-389.

1907. Tiwari, K.C. and Tiwari, V.P. "Some important medicinal plants of the tropical, subtropical and temperate region of Siang, Sabansiri and Tirap districts of Arunachal Pradesh". In Ethnobotany and medicinal plants of Indian sub-continent, edited by J.K. Maheshwari, Jodhpur, India Scientific Publishers, 2000.

1908. Tiwari, K.C., Joshi, G.C., Tiwari, V.P. and Tiwari, R.N. "Uttrakhand Himalaya Me Pashu Chikitsa Me Sthaniy Zadhi Butiyaon Ka Upyog". In Proceedings of National Symposium (July 6-7, 1998), on Constraints and Opportunities in Himalayan Region edited by P.C. Herbola, Indian Veterinary Research Institute, Mukteshwar, Kumaun (Nainital), U.P. pp. 129-135. [Hindi]

1909. Tiwari, K.C., Majumdar, R. and Bhattacharjee, S. "Folklore claims on medicines and treatments from Assam". *Bulletin of Medico-ethno-botanical Research*, Vol. 1, 1980, pp. 166-178.

1910. Tiwari, K.C., Majumdar, R. and Bhattacharjee, S. "Folklore medicine from Assam and Arunachal Pradesh (District Tirap)". *Quarterly Journal of Drug Research*, Vol. 17, 1979, pp. 61-67.

1911. Tiwari, K.C., Majumdar, R. and Bhattacharjee, S. "Tribal medicines and treatment from district Siang of Arunachal Pradesh". *Bulletin of Medico-ethno-botanical Research,* Vol. 1, 1980, pp. 440-446.

1912. Tiwari, Lait and Agrawal, D. P. "Tribal Medicine: the Untapped Treasure". (http://www.infinityfoundation.com/mandala/t_es/t_es_agraw_tribal_frameset.htm)

1913. Tiwari, Lalit and Pande, P.C. "Indigenous veterinary practices of Darma valley of Pithoragarh district, Uttaranchal". *Indian Journal of Traditional Knowledge,* Vol. 5, No. 2, 2006, pp. 201-206.

1914. Tiwari, S.C. and Mahanta, Debajit "Ethnological observations on fermented food products of certain tribes of Arunachal Pradesh". *Indian Journal of Traditional Knowledge,* Vol. 6, No. 1, 2007, pp. 106-110.

1915. Tiwari, U.L., Kotia, A. and Rawat, G.S. "Medico-ethnobotany of Monpas in Tawang and West Kaming districts of Arunachal Pradesh, India". *Pleione*, Vol. 3, No. 1, 2009, pp. 1-8.

1916. Tomar, Amit "Folk medicinal uses of plant roots from Meerut district", Uttar Pradesh". *Indian Journal of Traditional Knowledge,* Vol. 8, No. 2, 2009, pp. 298-301.

1917. Tribedi, G.N., Kayal, R.N. and Chaudhuri, H. N. Rai "Some medicinal plants of Mayurbhanj (Orissa)". *Bulletin of the Botanicl Survey of India,* Vol. 24, 1982, pp. 114-120.

1918. Tribhuwan, Robin and Peters, Preeti, "Medico-Ethnobiology of the Kathkaris and Thakurs". *Tribal Research Bulletin,* Vol. XIV, No.1, 1992, March, TRTI, Pune.

1919. Tribhuwan, Robin D. "Health of Primitive Tribes". Discover Publishing House, New Delhi, 2004, p. 186.

1920. Tribhuwan, Robin D. and Sherry, Karen "Health medicine and nutrition of the tribals". 2004, p. 66.

1921. Tripathi, G. "Indigenous knowledge and traditional practices of some Himalayan medicinal plants". In Himalayan Medicinal Plants: Potential and Prospects edited by S.S. Samant, U. Dhar and L. M.S. Palni, Gyanodaya Prakasan, Nainital. 2001, pp. 151-157.

1922. Tripathi, Hema, Mandape, M. K. and Kunzu, O. N. "Traditional wisdom of rural people about primary healthcare of children". *Indian Journal of Traditional Knowledge,* Vol. 3, No. 3, 2004, pp. 314-324.

1923. Tripathi, S. C. and Srivastava, Manjulla "Ethnomedicinal flora of euphorbiaceae used dermatological problems". *Indian Journal of Traditional Knowledge,* Vol. 9, No. 2, 2010, pp. 318-320.

1924. Tripathi, Sunil and Goel, Anil K. "Ethnobotanical Diversity of Zingiberaceae in North- Eastern India". *Ethnobotany,* Vol.13, No. 1-2, 2001, pp. 67-79.

1925. Tripathy, Basudev and Choudhury, B. C. "A review of sea turtle exploitation with special reference to Orissa, Andhra Pradesh and Lakshadweep Island, India". *Indian Journal of Traditional Knowledge,* Vol. 6, No. 2, 2007, pp. 285-291.

1926. Troisi, J. "Tribal religion: Religious beliefs and practices among the Santals". New Delhi, Manohar publications.1979.

1927. Tyagi, D. "Tribal Health in Anthropological Perspective". *Bulletin of the Department of Anthropology, Dibrugarh University*, Vol. 25, 2002, pp. 35-42.

1928. Udayan, P.S., George, Satheesh, and Balachandran, Indira "Ethnomedicine of the chellipale community of Namakkal district, Tamil Nadu". *Indian Journal of Traditional Knowledge,* Vol. 4, No. 4, 2005, pp. 437-442.

1929. Udayan, P.S., George, Satheesh, Tushar, K.V. and Balachandran, Indira "Ethnomedicine of Malapandaram tribes of Achenkovil forest of Kollam district, Kerala". *Indian Journal of Traditional Knowledge,* Vol. 6, No. 4, 2007, pp. 569-573.

1930. Udayan, P.S., Harinarayanan, M.K. and Tushar, K.V. "Some common plants used Kurichiar tribe of Tirunelli forest, Wayananad district, Kerala in medicine and other traditional". *Indian Journal of Traditional Knowledge,* Vol. 7, No. 2, 2008, pp. 250-255.

1931. Udayan, P.S., Satheesh, George, Thushar, K.V. and Balachandran, Indira "Ethnomedicine of chellipale community of Nammakkal district, Tamil Nadu Indian". *Indian Journal of Traditional Knowledge,* Vol. 4, No. 4, 2005, pp. 437-442.

1932. Umadevi, S.; Mohanta, G.P. and Manavalan, R. "Screening of folklore claim of Scaevola frutescens Krause". *Indian Journal of Traditional Knowledge,* Vol. 5, No. 4, 2006, pp. 531-536.

1933. Umapriya, T. and others "Ethnobotany of Irular tribe in Palamalai Hills, Coimbatore, Tamil Nadu". *Indian Journal of Natural Products and Resources,* Vol. 2, No. 2, 2011, pp. 250-255.

1934. Ummachan, M., Saini, Vimal and Sangeeta "Madhya Pradesh ki janjatiyo ki ausadhiya". *Jeevaniya*, Vol. 6, No. 1-2, 1995, p. 46. [Hindi]

1935. Uniyal, Bhagwati "Utilization of medicinal plants by the rural women of Kullu, Himachal Pradesh". *Indian Journal of Traditional Knowledge,* Vol. 2, No. 4, 2003, pp. 366-370.

1936. Uniyal, M.R. "A preliminary study of medicinal plants from Suru valley in Ladakh". *Bulletin of Medico-Ethno-Botanical Research*, Vol. 2, 1981, pp. 316-326.

1937. Uniyal, M.R. "Medicinal flora of Garhwal Himalaya". Sri Baidyanath Ayurved Bhawan Pvt. Ltd., Nagpur, 1989.

1938. Uniyal, M. R. "Medicinal plants collected from Bhilangana Valley during 1963-1964". *Sachitra Ayurved*, Vol. 17, 1964, pp. 365-368.

1939. Uniyal, M.R. "Medicinal plants of Bhagirathi valley laying in Uttarkashi Forest Division". *Indian Forester*, Vol. 94, 1968, pp. 407-420.

1940. Uniyal, M.R. "Parvatiya parisar me jalvau ke anusar jari-booti utpadan". Proceeding of All India Ayurvedia Congress, New Delhi, Ayurveda, Vol. 7, 1993, pp. 9-18. [Hindi]

1941. Uniyal, M.R. "Uttarakhand Vanaushadi Darshika". Centre Council for Research in Indian Medicine and Homeopathy, New Delhi, 1977. [Hindi]

1942. Uniyal, M.R. and Billore, K.V. "Tylophora hirsula wt. an indigenous drug for inducing abortion". *Journal of Research Indian Medicine*, Vol. 8, No. 1, 1973, p. 95

1943. Uniyal, M.R. and Chauhan, N.S. "Medicinal plant of Uhal valley in Kangra forest division, Himachal Pradesh". *Journal of Research Indian Medicine*, Vol. 4, No. 3, 1971, pp. 287-299.

1944. Uniyal, M.R. and Chauhan, N.S. "Traditionally important medicinal plants of Kangra valley in Dharamshala forest circle H. P.". *Journal of Indian Medical Research,* Vol. 8, 1973, pp. 7-85.

1945. Uniyal, M.R. and Issar, R.K. "Commercially important medicinal plants of Kanatal forest division Tehri Garhwal". *Indian Forming*, Vol. 93, 1967, pp. 107-114.

1946. Uniyal, M.R. and Joshi, G.C. "Cancer ke upchar mai paramparagat ausadhi bichu grass". *Sachitra Ayurved,* May 1991, pp. 719-720. [Hindi]

1947. Uniyal, M.R. and Joshi, G.C. "Historical view of the basic principal of the identification of the controversial drugs problems and suggestions". *Sachitra Ayurved,* January, 1993, pp. 531-536.

1948. Uniyal, M.R.and Joshi, G.C."Traditionally used family planning drug Babila Ghass from Garhwal Himalaya". *Sachitra Ayurved,* October 1986, pp. 198-400.

1949. Uniyal, M.R. and Misra, O.P. "Indigenous and traditional medicines in veterinary". *Sachitra Ayurved*, Vol. 29, No. 12, 1977, pp. 911-917.

1950. Uniyal, M.R. and R.K. Issar. "Commercially and traditionally important medicinal plants in Mandakini Valley of Uttar Khand Himalaya". *Journal of Research Indian Medicine*, Vol. 4, 1969, pp. 83-96.

1951. Uniyal, M.R., Tiwary, J., Chaubey, S.N. and Dixit, R.S. "Some medicinal plants as minor forest products in India". *Nagarjun*, Vol. 22, No. 5, 1979, pp. 114-117.

1952. Uniyal, Maya Ram "Hemkund evam Bhyundar Ghati ki Jadi- Bootiyan". *Himalaya Man and Nature*, Vol. 14, No. 10, 1991, pp. 25-27.

1953. Uniyal, S.K., Singh, K.N., Jamwal, P., Lal, B. "Traditional use of medicinal plants among the tribal communities of Chhota Bhangal, Western Himalaya". *Journal of Ethnobiology and Ethnomedicine,* Vol. 2, No.14, 2006.

1954. Unni, B.G., Goswami, Manoshi and Kakoty, Yelena "Indigenous knowledge of silkworm cultivation and its utilization in north eastern region of India". *Indian Journal of Traditional Knowledge,* Vol. 8, No. 1, 2009, pp. 70-74.

1955. Unnithan-Kumar, Maya "Midwives among Others: Knowledges of Healing and the Politics of Emotions Rajasthan, Northwest India". In The Daugthers of Hariti: Childbirth and Female Healers in South and Southeast Asia, edited by Santi Rozario and Geoffrey Samuel, London, Routledge, 2002, pp. 109-129.

1956. Unnithan-Kumar, Maya "Spirits of the womb: Migration,

reproductive choice and healing in Rajasthan". *Contributions to Indian Sociology*, Vol. 37, No, 1-2, 2003, pp. 163-188.

1957. Upadhya, Vinayak and others "Digital database on ethno-medicinal plants of Western Ghats". *Current Science*, Vol. 99, No. 12, 2010, pp. 1658-1659.

1958. Upadhyay, A.S., Kumbhojkar, M.S. and Kulkarni, V. "Ethno-medico botany of some sacred plants of Western Maharashtra". *Ethnobotany,* Vol. 9, 1997, pp. 65-68.

1959. Upadhyay, Ravi and Chauhan, S. V. S. "Ethnobotanical observations on Koya tribe of Gundala Mandal of Khammam district, Andhra Pradesh". *Ethnobotany,* Vol. 12, No. 1-2, 2009, pp. 93-99.

1960. Upadhyay, Ruchi and Singh, Jaswant "Ethno-medicinal uses of plants from Tikri Forest of Gonda district (U.P.)". *Ethnobotany,* Vol. 17, No. 1-2, 2005, pp. 167-170.

1961. Upadhye, A.S. and Kulkarni, D.K. "Traditional Phytotherapy for Insect Bites among the tribals in Western Maharashtra". *Ethnobotany,* Vol. 16, No. 1-2, 2004, pp. 59-61.

1962. Upadhye, A. S., Kumbhojkar, M.S. and Kulkarni, D.K. "Ethno-Medico-Botany of some sacred plants of Western Maharashtra". *Ethnobotany,* Vol. 9, No. 1-2, 1997, pp. 65-68.

1963. Upadhye, A., Kumbhojkar, M.S. and Vartak, V. D. "Observations on wild plants used in folk medicine in the rural areas of the Kolhapur district". *Ancient Science Life,* Vol. 6, 1986, pp. 119-121.

1964. Upadhye, Anuradha and Kumbhojkar, M.S. "Ethnobotany of genus Sterculia L. from India". In Ethnobotany and medicinal plants of Indian Sub-continent, edited by J.K. Maheshwari, Jodhpur, India Scientific Publishers, 2000.

1965. Upadhye, Anuradha S., Vartak, V.D. and Kumbhojkar, M.S. "Ethno-Medico-Botanical Studies in Western Maharashtra, India". *Ethnobotany,* Vol. 6, No. 1-2, 1994, pp. 25-31.

1966. Upreti, D.K. "Studies in Indian ethnolichenology". In Ethnobiology in Human Welfare edited by S.K. Jain, Deep Publication, New Delhi. 1996, pp. 413-414.

1967. Upreti, D.K. and Negi, H.R. "Folk use of Thamnolia vermicularis (Swartz) Ach. in Schaerer in Lata village of Nanda Devi biosphere reserve". *Ethnobotany,* Vol. 8, 1996, pp. 83-86.

1968. Vaidya, Bhagwan Dash and Ramaswamy, Suhasini "Ayurveda: the science of traditional Indian medicine". Lustre Press, New Delhi, 1998, p. 84.

1969. Vaidya, M. Radhika and Balsubramanian, A. V. (eds.) "Mother and child care in traditional medicine (2 pts.)" . Madras, LSPSS, 1990, p. 81-78.

1970. Valiathan, M. S. "Ayurveda: Putting the house in order". Science, Vol. 90, No. 1, 2006, pp. 5-6.

1971. Vannucci, M. "Sacred groves or holi forests". In Concpt of space ancient and modern edited by Kapila Vatsyayan, Abhinav, New Delhi, 1991, pp. 323-331.

1972. Varghese, Earaplackal, Jain, S.K. and Bose, Niranjan "A quantitative approach to establish the Efficacy of Herbal Remedies: a case study on the Kharias". *Ethnobotany,* Vol. 5, No. 1-2, 1993, pp. 149-154.

1973. Varier's, Vaidyaratnam P.S. "Indian medicinal plants: A compendium of 500 species (in 4 Vols.)". Madras, Orient Longman, 1994.

1974. Varma, Daya R. "From witchcraft to allopathy: Uninterrupted journey of medical science". *Economic and Political Weekly,* Vol. 41, No. 33, 2006, pp. 3605-3611.

1975. Varma, S. K. "Comparative studies of folk drugs of tribals of Chotanagpur and Santhal Parganas of Bihar India". Ethnobiology in Human welfare: IV Inter Congress of Ethnobiology, Lucknow (India), 1994, p. 77.

1976. Varma, S.K. and Pandey, A.K. "Ethnobotany notes on certain medicinal plants used by the tribals of Lohardaga district Bihar". *Journal of Economic and Taxonomic Botany,* Vol. 14, No. 2, 1990, pp. 329-333.

1977. Varma, S.K., Srivastava, D.K. and Sharma, R.K. "Tapping some medicinal plants for tribal development in Santhal Pargana". *Journal Regional Studies*, Vol. 1, No. 2, 1986, pp. 85-92.

1978. Vartak, V. D. "Some edible wild plants from the hilly region of the Poona district, Bombay State". *Journal of Bombay Natural History Society*, Vol. 56, 1959, pp. 455-458.

1979. Vartak, V. D. "Studies of ethnobotany of Maharashtra and Goa". *Tribal Research Bulletin*, Vol. 4, No. 2, 1982, pp. 9-10.

1980. Vartak, V. D. and Mandavgane, R. "Enumeration of medicinal plants form tribals of Maharashtra". *Journal of University of Poona Science Technology*, Vol. 54, 1981, pp. 91-99.

1981. Ved Prakash, and Mehrotra, B. N. "Unrecorded traditional medicines-1". *Ancient Science of Life*, Vol. 8, No. 2, 1988, pp. 110-112.

1982. Vedavathy, S. "Herbal Folk Medicine of Yanadis of Andhra Pradesh". *Ethnobotany,* Vol. 8, No. 1-2, 1996, pp. 109-111.

1983. Vedavathy, S. "Scope and importance of traditional medicine". *Indian Journal of Traditional Knowledge,* Vol. 2, No. 3, 2003, pp. 236-239.

1984. Vedavathy, S. "Tribal medicine-the real alternative". *Indian Journal of Traditional Knowledge,* Vol. 1, No. 1, 2002, pp. 25- 31.

1985. Vedavathy, S., Mrudula, V., Sudhakar, A. and Siddhamma, T. "Tribal medicine of Andhra Pradesh". *Ancient Science of Life*, Vol. 18, No. 1, 1998, pp. 58-63.

1986. Vedavathy, S., Mrudula, V., Sudhakar, A. "Tribal medicine of Chittoor district, Andhra Pradesh". *Herbal Folklore Research Centre*, Tirupati, 1997, p. 165.

1987. Venkataraman, K. and Raju, R.R. Venkata "Folk Medicine from Gundlabrahmeswaram Wild-Life Sanctuary, Andhra Pradesh". *Ethnobotany,* Vol. 16, No. 1-2, 2004, pp. 33-39.

1988. Venkatraman, R. "A history of the Tamil Siddha cult". Ennes Publications, Madurai, 1990, p. 283.

1989. Venkatraman, R. "Medical Sociology in an Indian setting". New Delhi, Macmillan Company of India Limited, 1979.

1990. Venu Gopal, P.N. and Nanjunda, D.C. "Role of indigenous knowledge in the forest management of Betta and Koraga tribal women of Karnataka (India): reconsideration". *Man in India,* Vol. 35, No. 1-2, 2009, pp. 59-64.

1991. Venugopal K. and Raghunathan, K. "Medicobotanical-cum-ethnomedicinal survey of district Jhabua (M.P.)". *Centre Coun. Res. Ayur. Siddha Newsletter*, Vol. 4-5, 1982.

1992. Venugopal, S.N. "Management of common problems of ear, nose and throat in primary health care". Coimbatore, Lok Swasthya Parampara Samvardhan Samithi, p. 69.

1993. Verma, Archana K., Munesh Kumar and Rainer, W. Bussmann "Medicinal plants in an urban environment: The medicinal flora of Banares Hindu University, Varanasi Uttar Pradesh". *Journal of Ethnobiology and Ethnomedicine*, Vol. 3, No. 35, 2007.

1994. Verma, Arti, Singhal, Asha and Singh, Dheeraj "Local health wisdom of rural women using medicinal plants". *Indian Journal of Traditional Knowledge,* Vol. 9, No. 2, 2010, pp. 289-293.

1995. Verma, Chiralekha, Bhatia, Shashi and Srivastava, Shuchi "Traditional medicine of the Nicobarese". *Indian Journal of Traditional Knowledge,* Vol. 9, No. 4, 2010, pp. 779-785.

1996. Verma, P., Khan, A.A. and Singh, K.K. "Traditional phytotherapy among the Baiga tribe of Shahdol district of Madhya Pradesh, India." *Ethnobotany,* Vol. 7, No. 1-2, 1995, pp. 69-73.

1997. Verma, R.L. "Indian –Arab relations in medical sciences". In History of Medicine in India, edited by P.V. Sharma New Delhi, Indian National Science Academy 1992, pp. 465-484.

1998. Verma, Saroj and Chauhan, N. S. "Indigenous medicinal plants knowledge of Kunihar forest division, district Solan". *Indian Journal of Traditional Knowledge,* Vol. 6, No. 3, 2007, pp. 494-497.

1999. Verma, Saroj and Chauhan, N.S. "Studies on Ethno-Medico-Botany of Kunihar Forest Division, district Solan (H.P)". *Ethnobotany,* Vol. 18, No. 1-2, 2006, pp. 160-165.

2000. Vidyasagar, G.M. and Prashantkumar, P. "Traditional herbal remedies for gynaecological disorder in women of Bidar district, Karnataka, India". *Fitoterapia*, Vol. 78, 2007, pp. 48-51.

2001. Vijayalakshmi, K. "Mrgayurveda Indian animal science (in

2 parts)". Madras, Lok Swasthya Parampara Samvardhan Samithi, 1994, p. 68-71.

2002. Vijayendra, B.R. and Bhat, H.K. "Ethnomedicine among the Jenu Kuruba of Karnataka". In Tribal health and medicines, edited by A.K. Kalla and P.C. Joshi, New Delhi: Concept Publishing Co., 2004, pp. 391-402.

2003. Vinay Kumar "Jaunsar Bavar Janjati ke ajube chikitsa Paddhati". *Vanyajati*, Vol. 52, No. 4, 2004, pp. 40-48. [Hindi]

2004. Vineet, Singh, Dubey, Priyanka, and Srivastava, Sharad "Botanical standardization of the Jatamansi, their substitute and adulterant species". *Indian Journal of Traditional Knowledge,* Vol. 10, No. 4, 2011, pp. 599-603.

2005. Vishwanathan, M.B., Kumar, E.H. Prem and Ramesh, N. "Ethnomedicines of Kanis in Kalakkad-Mundanthurai Tiger Reserve, Tamil Nadu". *Ethnobotany*, Vol. 13, No. 1-2, 2001, pp. 60-66.

2006. Viswanathan, M.B. "Ethnobotany of the Malayalis in North Arcot district, Tamil Nadu, India". *Ethnobotany*, Vol. 9, No. 1-2, 1997, pp. 77-79.

2007. Viswanathan, M.V, Raja, D. Karpaga and Khanna, S. Durai "Siddha way to cure chikungunya". *Indian Journal of Traditional Knowledge,* Vol. 7, No. 2, 2008, pp. 345-346.

2008. Viswanathan, M.V., Unnikrishnan, P.M. and Komatsu, Katsuko "A brief introduction to ayurvedic system of medicine and some of its problems". *Indian Journal of Traditional Knowledge,* Vol. 2, No. 2, 2003, pp. 159-169.

2009. Vohora, S.B. "Animal origin drugs used in unani medicine". New Delhi, Vikas, 1979, p. 137.

2010. Wagh, Vijay V., Jain, Ashok K. and Kadel, Chitralekha "Ethnomedicinal plants used for curing dysentery and diarrhoea by tribals of Jhabua District (Madhya Pradesh)". *Indian Journal of Natural Products and Resources,* Vol. 2, No. 2, 2011, pp. 256-260.

2011. Wainwright, Milton "Moulds in folk medicine". *Folklore*, Vol. 100, No. 2, 1989, pp. 162-166.

2012. Warman, C.K. "Trees of India: Medicinal, commercial, religious and ornamental: a colour atlas". New Delhi, CBS, 1999, p. 246.

2013. Warren, D.M., David Brokensha and Slikkerveer, L. Jan "Indigenous knowledge systems: the cultural dimension of development". London, Kegan Paul International, 1992.

2014. Weiss, Richard S. "Recipes for immortality: Healing, religion, and community in South India". Oxford University Press, 2009, p. 272.

2015. Wellin, E. "Theoretical orientations in Medical Anthropology: continuity and change over the past half century". In Culture, Disease and healing: studies in medical anthropology, edited by D. Landy, London, Collier Macmillan Publishers, 1977.

2016. Williams, L. A.D. "Ethnomedicine". *West Indian Medicinal Journal*, Vol. 55, No. 4, 2006, pp. 215-216.

2017. Wilsanad, V., Varghese, Preema and Rajitha, P. "Therapeutics of insects and insect products in South Indian traditional medicine". *Indian Journal of Traditional Knowledge,* Vol. 6, No.4, 2007, pp. 563- 568.

2018. Wilsanand, V. "Utilization of termite, Odontotermes formosanus by tribes of South India in medicine and food". *Indian Journal of Natural Products and Resources*, Vol. 8, No. 1, 2009, pp. 73-76.

2019. Winker, C.W. "The emergence of biomedical anthropology and its implications for the future". *American Journal of Physical Anthropology*, Vol. 64, 1984, pp. 141-46.

2020. Wirsing, Rolf L. "The health of traditional societies and the effects of Acculturation". *Current Anthropology*, Vol. 26, No. 3, 1985.

2021. Wolff, Robert J. "Modern medicine and traditional culture: Confrontation on the Malay Peninsula". *Human Organization*, Vol. 24, No. 4, 1986.

2022. Wood, Corinne "The Traditional Healer". In Human Sickness and Health: A Biocultural View, Palo Alto, CA: Mayfield Publishers.1979, pp. 291-334.

2023. Woodward, E. F. "Literature searches for uses of new botanical drugs". *Advances in Chemistry Series*, Vol. 16, 1956, pp. 162-167.

2024. Worsley, Peter "Non-Western Medical Systems". *Annual Review of Anthropology*, Vol. 11, 1982, pp. 315-348.

2025. Xaxa, Virginius "Transformation of Tribes in India: Terms of Discourse". *Economic and Political Weekly*, Vol. 34, No. 24, 1999, pp. 1519-1524.

2026. Yadaiah, G., Parul Joshi, Bindiya, Oza "Traditional knowledge of wild medicinal plants of Baria forest division, Dahod District, Gujarat state". *Indian Forester*, Vol. 137, No. 7, pp. 814-821.

2027. Yadav, J.P., Kumar, Suresh and Siwach, Priyanka "Folk medicine used in gynecological and other related problems by rural population of Haryana". *Indian Journal of Traditional Knowledge,* Vol. 5, No. 3, 2006, pp. 323-326.

2028. Yamashita, Tsutomu and Manohar, P. Ram "Memoirs of Vaidyas: The Lives and Practices of Traditional Medical Doctors in Kerala". *Indian Journal of Indian Medicine*, Vol. 4, No. 1, 2011.

2029. Yesodharan, K. and Sujana, K. A. "Ethnomedicinal knowledge among Malamalasar tribe Parambikulam wildlife sanctuary, Kerala". *Indian Journal of Traditional Knowledge,* Vol. 6, No.3, 2007, pp. 481- 485.

2030. Young, A. "Some implications of medical beliefs and practices for social anthropology". *American Anthropologist*, Vol. 78, 1976, pp. 5-24.

2031. Yumkham, S. D. and Singh, P. K. "Less known ferns and fern-allies of Manipur with ethnobotanic uses". *Indian Journal of Traditional Knowledge,* Vol. 10, No. 2, 2011, pp. 287-291.

2032. Yumnam, J.Y. and Tripathi, O.P. "Traditional knowledge of eating raw plants by the Meitei of Manipur as medicine/ nutrient supplement in their diet". *Indian Journal of Traditional Knowledge,* Vol. 11, No. 1, 2012, pp. 45-50.

2033. Zafar, Rasheeduz "Medicinal plants of India". Delhi, CBS, 1994, p. 132.

2034. Zutshi, Usha and others "New utilization of some indigenous drugs". Paper present at the National Symposium on the Development of Indigenous Drugs in India, New Delhi, April 8-10, 1988.

Keyword/ Subject Index

C

D

F

H

O

P

S

T

V

Title Index